UNDERSTANDING NURSING AND HEALTHCARE RESEARCH

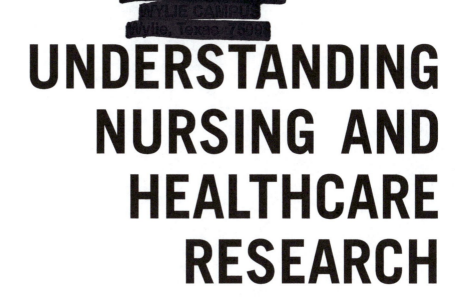

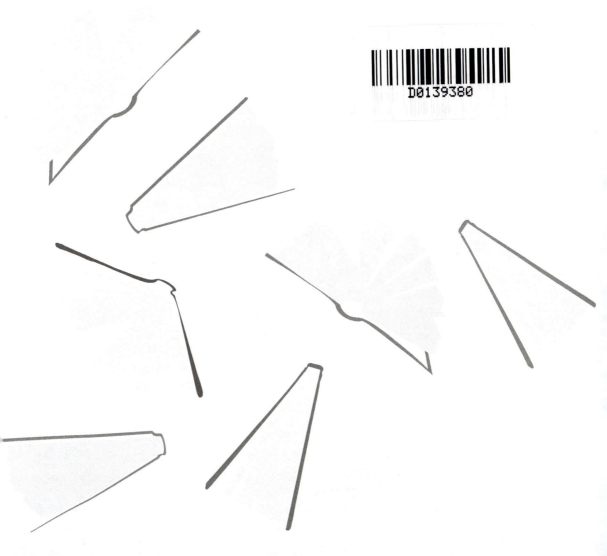

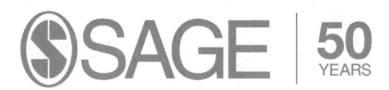

SAGE was founded in 1965 by Sara Miller McCune to support the dissemination of usable knowledge by publishing innovative and high-quality research and teaching content. Today, we publish more than 750 journals, including those of more than 300 learned societies, more than 800 new books per year, and a growing range of library products including archives, data, case studies, reports, conference highlights, and video. SAGE remains majority-owned by our founder, and after Sara's lifetime will become owned by a charitable trust that secures our continued independence.

Los Angeles | London | Washington DC | New Delhi | Singapore

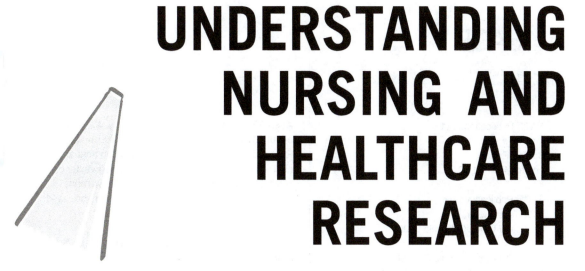

UNDERSTANDING NURSING AND HEALTHCARE RESEARCH

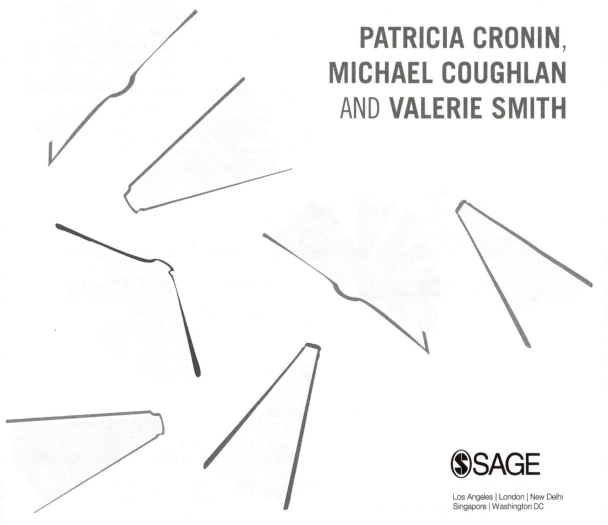

PATRICIA CRONIN, MICHAEL COUGHLAN AND VALERIE SMITH

⑤SAGE

Los Angeles | London | New Delhi
Singapore | Washington DC

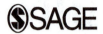

Los Angeles | London | New Delhi
Singapore | Washington DC

SAGE Publications Ltd
1 Oliver's Yard
55 City Road
London EC1Y 1SP

SAGE Publications Inc.
2455 Teller Road
Thousand Oaks, California 91320

SAGE Publications India Pvt Ltd
B 1/I 1 Mohan Cooperative Industrial Area
Mathura Road
New Delhi 110 044

SAGE Publications Asia-Pacific Pte Ltd
3 Church Street
#10-04 Samsung Hub
Singapore 049483

Editor: Becky Taylor
Associate Editor: Emma Milman
Production editor: Katie Forsythe
Copyeditor: Bryan Campbell
Proofreader: Danielle Ray
Indexer: Caroline Eley
Marketing manager: Camille Richmond
Cover design: Naomi Robinson
Typeset by: C&M Digitals (P) Ltd, Chennai, India

At SAGE we take sustainability seriously. We print most of our products in the UK. These are produced using FSC papers and boards. We undertake an annual audit on materials used to ensure that we monitor our sustainability in what we are doing. When we print overseas, we ensure that sustainable papers are used, as measured by the Egmont grading system.

Library of Congress Control Number: 2014939625

British Library Cataloguing in Publication data

A catalogue record for this book is available from the British Library

ISBN 978-1-4462-4100-4
ISBN 978-1-4462-4101-1 (pbk)

At SAGE we take sustainability seriously. Most of our products are printed in the UK using FSC papers and boards. When we print overseas we ensure sustainable papers are used as measured by the Egmont grading system. We undertake an annual audit to monitor our sustainability.

Contents

List of Figures and Tables

Figures

Tables

About the Authors

Patricia Cronin is an Assistant Professor in the School of Nursing and Midwifery, Trinity College Dublin prior to which she worked at City University, London. She has been involved in healthcare education for 20 years. Her clinical background is in surgical and gastrointestinal nursing, which she teaches at undergraduate level. She has a special interest in enabling students to engage in research and theory and these areas form the focus of her postgraduate teaching. She has published widely, co-authoring three books and has written book chapters and journal articles related to clinical skills, gastrointestinal nursing, research and theory.

Qualifications: PhD, MSc, BSc Nursing & Education, DipN (Lond), RN.

Michael Coughlan is an Assistant Professor in the School of Nursing, Trinity College Dublin, where he has worked since 2002. He is a Registered Nurse Tutor and has been involved in nurse education for over 20 years. He has a wide experience in guiding and supervising students undertaking literature reviews and research studies at both an undergraduate and postgraduate level. His interests include research, and haematology and oncology nursing and he has a number of publications in these areas, including co-authoring a book on undertaking literature reviews.

Qualifications: BNS, MEd., RPN, RGN, RNT.

Valerie Smith is a part-time Assistant Professor in the School of Nursing and Midwifery, Trinity College Dublin and a part-time Research Fellow in the School of Nursing and Midwifery, National University of Ireland, Galway. She is a Registered Midwife, Nurse Tutor and General Nurse and has been involved in healthcare education and research since 2005. She currently leads modules on research evidence for practice, supervises and mentors students at undergraduate and postgraduate level and facilitates workshops on research methods, in particular, systematic review methodology. She has published widely in the area of maternity care and research methods, reviews for six international healthcare journals, and is an associate editor for the BMC Pregnancy and Childbirth journal.

Qualifications: PhD, MSc, BSc (Hons) Midwifery, PGDip (Stats), PGDip (CHSE), BNS, RGN, RM, RNT.

About the Companion Website

Visit the companion website at https://study.sagepub.com/cronin to find a range of teaching and learning material for lecturers and students, including the following.

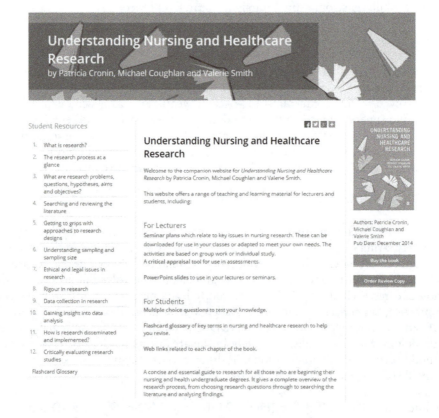

For Lecturers

Seminar plans which relate to key issues in nursing research. These can be downloaded for use in your classes or adapted to meet your own needs. The activities are based on group work or individual study.

PowerPoint slides to use in your lectures or seminars.

For Students

Free online readings to use as examples of research. These are indicated by the icon in the text.

Multiple choice questions to test your knowledge.

Flashcard glossary of key terms in nursing and healthcare research to help you revise.

Web links related to each chapter of the book.

Critical appraisal tool for use in assessments.

1

What is Research?

Introduction

This book is designed as an introductory text that will facilitate your understanding of research. Undertaking research is a skilled activity and while it is desirable that practitioners engage in research this is not the purpose of this book. This book is focussed on introducing you to research so that you can become research aware. Being research aware is about developing the skills that will enable you to read and understand research reports. While this may seem straightforward, understanding research means possessing the skills to make judgements about the quality of that research and determining if the findings are sufficiently credible to warrant implementation in practice. In order to do this you must know about each step of the research process and be able to decide if the study has been conducted in the way it should have been. Understanding research is a fundamental and necessary skill for all healthcare practitioners because we have to be sure that the care and treatment of those in our care is based on the best available evidence. As will be shown further on in this chapter, research evidence is a key element of evidence-based practice. Much of the content will be directed at what is known as 'applied' research, that is, research that has application to clinical practice.

This introductory chapter sets the scene for subsequent chapters. This is because we believe if you have some insight into the history of research you are more likely to understand why it has developed in the way it has. Some of the concepts that are presented will be new to you and it may take several readings to understand the more complex of these. The chapter begins by offering a brief definition of research. Subsequent sections outline the relationship between research and knowledge, research and theory and research and practice. The chapter concludes by exploring the importance of becoming research aware and how this is ultimately related to research utilisation in practice.

☑ **Learning Outcomes** ☑

By the end of this chapter you should be able to:

- Explain what is meant by research
- Outline the relationship between research and knowledge
- Describe how theory and research are related
- Summarise how research is important for clinical practice
- Identify what it means to be research aware.

What is Research?

The word 'research' originates in the Old French 'recercher' which means to 'seek out, search closely'. It appeared in the English language in the seventeenth century and was taken to mean 'a careful search for facts'. Although we commonly use the word in our everyday language, for example, 'I researched the options for our holiday' its primary usage is in the world of science where its meaning remains closely linked with its original seventeenth century conception. Contemporary research can be said to be concerned with examining, looking closely or scrutinising an issue of interest for the purpose of better understanding. This may ultimately lead to a refinement, validation or refutation of current knowledge and/or the creation of new knowledge. Research in this context is referred to as empirical research and is synonymous with the use of a structured method. There are two key points that emerge here. The first is concerned with the question of what constitutes knowledge and the second is about the use of a structured method.

Knowledge and Research

In considering the first point, the study of knowledge, its history, its origins and the criteria for what counts as knowledge is a branch of philosophy known as 'epistemology'. Epistemological questions such as 'what is knowledge' and 'what is truth' have challenged and even vexed philosophers since the time of early Greek philosophers such as Plato and Aristotle (Steup, 2012). There have been sharp disagreements about what knowledge is and what counts as knowledge and seeking answers to these questions has been and remains fraught with difficulty.

However, what has emerged is an agreement that there are different types of knowledge. Although we accept much of what we know as a given and consequently do not afford it much thought, there is little doubt that we all know many things about the world in which we live. Moreover, our knowledge is changing and expanding all the time depending on what we read, what we experience or what we are told. We not only know *about* people, places and things, we know *how to do* things such as ride a bicycle, play a piano, dance, read and sing. We also experience the world and come to know things such as sadness, happiness and pain through those experiences. All of these constitute different kinds of knowledge that make up all of what we know.

These types of knowledge have been variously classified but most commonly include propositional, procedural and personal knowledge. Propositional knowledge or 'knowledge that' is that knowledge we have when we say that 'such and such is the case'. Propositional knowledge includes the knowledge of theories, facts and laws. For example, when we say we know each key on a piano denotes a musical note we are speaking of propositional knowledge.

However, knowing this does not mean that we possess the necessary skills to play the piano. The knowledge of *how* to do something is signified as procedural knowledge and can only be developed by learning through doing. Thus, exposure and experience is central to developing procedural knowledge although it is important to note that procedural knowledge may entail some propositional knowledge.

The third type of knowledge identified by epistemologists is personal knowing, which has also been described as 'knowledge by acquaintance' and is the knowledge that we have by virtue of having experienced something. For instance, we can only know pain by having experienced it. However, for it to be considered knowledge, we must be able to determine that what we are experiencing is indeed pain and for this we need to have some propositional knowledge of the concept of pain. As with procedural knowledge it seems that personal knowledge also involves possessing some propositional knowledge.

Consider the three types of knowledge above in respect of the activity of recording of a person's blood pressure. See if you can identify:

- The propositional knowledge (theories) that underpins the activity, i.e. why is it done, what does it tell us and why is that important?
- The procedural knowledge that you would need to be able to complete the activity. How do you acquire this knowledge?
- Any personal knowledge you have regarding the activity, e.g. have you had your blood pressure recorded and what do you think you learned from this experience?

ACTIVITY 1.1

If, as can be seen from the above outline, procedural knowledge is associated with learning from doing and personal knowledge arises from our experiences of the world, how do we acquire propositional knowledge? Even though philosophers concerned with epistemology acknowledge procedural and personal knowledge, their primary focus is on propositional knowledge and how it is developed. Philosophically speaking there are two opposing traditions about our sources of knowledge that are known as rationalism and empiricism.

Rationalism essentially argues that propositional knowledge comes to us through the use of reason. The basic premise is that our minds generate knowledge because of our ability to think. Philosophers such as Descartes who was a key figure in rationalism believed that we could not trust what our senses were telling us. He argued that because there were so many ways of interpreting reality we could only be sure of our own thinking. His famous phrase 'I think, therefore I am' comes from this belief.

Conversely, empiricism is located in the belief that we are born with a 'tabula rasa' (blank slate) and our knowledge is derived from our experiences of the world. The notion of a 'tabula rasa' was first proposed by Aristotle and subsequently developed by a group of philosophers including the prominent English philosopher John Locke. He argued that our experiences consist of two parts, namely sensation and reflection. Our sensations happen through our senses of sight, hearing, taste, touch and smell and reflection is about how we interpret those experiences, which suggests that reasoning does play a part in how we make sense of things.

Nowadays, these positions would be seen to represent extremes and it would be unusual to find a philosopher who believes that knowledge is solely developed through reason or experience. Modern philosophy of science is less polarised and there is recognition that rationalism and empiricism both contribute to the development of propositional knowledge through the practical endeavour of undertaking research.

Philosophers are concerned about establishing the truth of things and in order to do this they had to develop methods that would help determine with as much certainty as possible if something was true. These methods varied depending on whether the philosopher was a rationalist or empiricist. For example, and as stated above, empiricism is concerned with the belief that knowledge comes from our experiences of the world. Therefore, the methods developed for establishing 'truth' are located in observing and measuring those experiences.

During the Renaissance and the Enlightenment period that followed, these approaches became the cornerstones of the methods used to establish the truth. Fundamentally, knowledge is amassed through repeated observation and measurement of particular instances of a phenomenon. The key approach to observing and measuring is the experiment where the purpose is to establish cause and effect and generalise the findings to the wider world. This process may begin to show general patterns, which ultimately result in building or generating theories that describe, explain or predict part of our world. Although this method, known as induction (bottom-up), has evolved and developed since the Enlightenment, characteristics such as measurement, the generalisation of findings to the wider world and the use of the experiment remain central to the work of researchers today.

The competing method, known as deduction (top-down) and located in rationalism and the work of Descartes works the other way and begins with a general principle, which is then applied to a specific situation. This method is also evident in contemporary research whereby researchers begin with a theory about some phenomenon. The theory may come from repeated observations about the phenomenon or topic of interest. It is then tested through research (see Figure 1.1). The researcher develops propositions (hypotheses) from the theory, which are then tested in specific situations. The outcome or the findings of the study will indicate whether the theory is valid or whether it can be refuted. This approach is broadly classified as theory testing.

Theory and Research

The important distinction between the two approaches outlined above is whether or not the researcher *begins* with a theory or *ends* with a theory. Regardless of which approach is taken or even if there is, as there are in some studies, a combination of both, the outcome

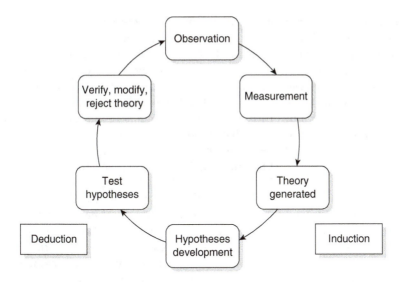

Figure 1.1   Inductive/deductive research cycle

is always about theory. Theories are those things that tie together all the propositional knowledge we have about a topic of interest and offer explanations for why something is the way it is. Thus, the ultimate aim of all scientific research is to devise theories that describe, explain, predict or control aspects of our world. The more the findings of research support the theory, the more certain we can be that it is true. Conversely, through research, theories can be found to be false and are rejected and in many cases replaced with alternative explanations that are a more accurate reflection of reality.

In many areas, competing theories exist and it is only with repeated research that one *may* emerge as having more explanatory value. For instance, there are a number of competing theories about why people commit crime. For the purposes of illustration two are mentioned here because of their quite different perspectives. The biological, genetic and evolution theory proposes that issues such as poor diet, mental illness, disorders of brain circuits are factors in whether or not somebody becomes involved in crime. Conversely, social learning theory argues that people develop a motivation to commit crime because of those with whom they associate. Determining which theory has more validity will depend, to some extent, on how much and what kind of evidence there is to support it.

While this may appear quite straightforward, there are factors that influence the type of research that is undertaken. For example, a biologist will undertake research that is directed at trying to establish if biology and genetics explain crime while a psychologist who supports social learning theory will strive to demonstrate that those with whom we associate is a motivating factor in committing crime. Either or both positions will only change when there is overwhelming evidence to support or refute a particular stance.

Even if it is ultimately shown that one theory has more explanatory value than another there are very few theories that are absolutely certain and they are always changing and evolving. Although simplified here, a good example of how theories evolve and change is the claim by Copernicus in the sixteenth century that the earth orbited the sun. While we might find it hard to comprehend today that this was ever in dispute, we should consider both the context in which the claim was made and the means that were available to verify the claim. Copernicus was an astronomer but he was only able to make observations of the sky with the naked eye as the telescope had not been invented. It was with its subsequent development that Galileo was able to confirm the accuracy of Copernicus' theory. Although there have been subsequent modifications of the theory, much of what Copernicus proposed has stood the test of time.

In terms of how readily Copernicus' theory was accepted, the context in which it was proposed is important. At the time, the Church in Rome had the power to determine what was accepted as theory or knowledge. Challenging its teachings, which were based on Aristotelian principles that the earth was static and the sun orbited it was a dangerous endeavour and for some led to charges of heresy and even death. Therefore, it was sometime after Copernicus' death that his theory was accepted.

There are some salient points to be noted in relation to this very brief discussion about theory and research. Primarily, it would be naïve of us to think that undertaking research and developing theories is context free. Members of a scientific community who undertake research tend to have collective beliefs and a common view of the world. What this means is that people who belong to the same community of scientists share beliefs about what constitutes knowledge, what theories they regard as valid and how research is or should be undertaken. Moreover, because of these commonly-held beliefs and views the research they conduct will likely serve to perpetuate that view or maintain the status quo. Kuhn (1970), a physicist, coined the term 'paradigm' to describe these underlying assumptions and the intellectual structure of scientific communities that drives research and development within them. So, if a researcher is a member of a community that subscribes to a biological view of why people commit crime then it is likely that he/she will also hold such a view.

The second point is related to what can be referred to as the prevailing view. While it is unlikely that modern day theorists and researchers would be burned at the stake, there is a legacy in terms of the notion that those who are in power or those who are seen to be powerful have the capacity to dictate and determine what counts as knowledge. Furthermore, those who are powerful influence what aspects of our lives deserve investigation. Therefore, while researchers may develop knowledge about topics they consider worthy, if it is not deemed to be so by powerful scientific communities it is unlikely to receive any attention.

The final point may seem self-evident but it is that knowledge development through research is facilitated or constrained by the means we have at our disposal. Remember Copernicus' lack of a telescope. Many of the research advances in the twentieth century have been facilitated by the phenomenal developments in technology. Our capacity for investigating phenomena of interest, the way in which we conduct research, how we manage the findings of research and our ability to disseminate those findings to a wide audience have been revolutionised.

Practice and Research

At this stage, you may be asking what all of this has to do with what we do as practitioners in healthcare. In healthcare practice, the underlying premise of our work is that we have a professional obligation to try to provide the best care possible based on the best available knowledge and evidence. Knowledge generated from research is one form of evidence and within the community of healthcare, research is undertaken to generate and test theories about health and illness with the aim of applying that knowledge for the ultimate benefit of those for whom we care.

In contemporary healthcare there is almost universal recognition from practitioners, managers and policy-makers that in order to deliver effective healthcare, scientific evidence is an essential element (Coughlan et al., 2013). This element, combined with the expertise of the clinician and the needs of the individual patient comprise clinical decision-making that is designed to introduce consistency in terms of care and treatment so that patient outcomes and quality of life can be improved. This model of clinical decision-making is known as evidence-based practice (EBP) (Sackett et al., 1996; Muir Gray, 2001).

The inclusion of sound scientific (research) evidence into clinical decision-making reduces the emphasis on what Guyatt et al. (2004: 390) described as 'unsystematic clinical experience and pathophysiological rationale'. In other words, external research evidence reduces the potential for practice based on individual preference or ritual that may not be in the patient's best interests.

This brings us to the question of what constitutes best research evidence. In this, the history of knowledge development has had a significant influence because characteristics of the scientific method alluded to earlier such as objectivity, measurement, generalisation, hypothesis testing and the use of the experiment are still considered to be central to the conduct of research that produces findings that are seen to be more reliable than research that does not contain them. Put more simply, the belief is that some research designs produce more reliable results than others. Thus, with the emergence of EBP, hierarchies of evidence have been developed.

In healthcare, much research is undertaken to find out what works best and these can be broadly classified as intervention studies. For these types of projects, the findings from randomised controlled trials (RCTs) (see Chapter 5) that are used to assess the effectiveness of clinical interventions, such as in the area of drugs or surgery, are generally considered to be the most reliable form of evidence. This is because in a randomised controlled trial the characteristics of the scientific method mentioned above are adopted to ensure that the results of the study can be attributed to the intervention being investigated as opposed to any other potential influence or variable. The less these characteristics are contained in a study the less reliable its findings are deemed to be. This is not to say that the findings of these other types of study are of no use but they are believed to be less 'certain'.

However, healthcare is complex, has a wide scope and is not just about clinical interventions. Therefore, other forms of research evidence are important in enabling us to gain a greater understanding of the illness experiences of patients and clients. For example, a randomised controlled trial can examine the effectiveness of a new medication but research evidence gained from qualitative studies is needed in order for us to determine how patients feel the medication impacts on their lives. Moreover, it could be that despite an intervention being clinically effective it may work differently or not at all depending on the individual, social, economic and environmental circumstances in which it is being implemented. Therefore, it is not appropriate to take the findings of a study and implement them without first determining how it works, how well it works, for whom it works and in what situation. What this means is that research evidence on its own is not sufficient for, and does not account for, the whole of clinical decision-making. This then speaks to the other two elements of EBP, namely, clinical expertise and the needs of the patient.

According to Gerrish (2010) clinical expertise is proficiency gained through experience. The inclusion of the word proficiency is important because as Rolfe (1999) states, the knowledge gained from experience may not always be used wisely or appropriately. Therefore, to have expertise means to be able to apply that knowledge 'wisely' to the care and treatment of patients.

Knowledge accumulated from experience is termed experiential knowledge and comprises the procedural and personal knowledge referred to earlier in this chapter. While there is some debate in the literature about whether experiential knowledge can constitute evidence (Hek & Moule, 2006; Rolfe & Gardner, 2006; Gerrish, 2010) it is clear that the experiential knowledge of the clinical expert is an essential element of EBP. Moreover, knowing the patient's needs and engaging with them to determine their preferences is fundamental. These three elements have an interdependent relationship that forms the whole of EBP with the underlying premise being that clinical decision-making should not be based exclusively on any one of the elements but on an amalgamation of all three.

While this model for clinical decision-making appears laudable there are a number of significant issues that impact on how research evidence as a component of EBP is utilised or translated into practice. Since as early as 1990 there have been a large number of publications in the healthcare literature addressing facilitators and barriers to research utilisation across a range of professions and settings (Bircumshaw, 1990; Parahoo, 2000; Hutchinson & Johnston, 2004; Milner et al., 2006; Thompson et al., 2008; Brown et al., 2010; Chien, 2010; Kocaman et al., 2010; Cobban & Profetto-McGrath, 2011; Lyons et al., 2011; Moreno-Casbas et al., 2011; Wangansteen et al., 2011; Christie et al., 2012; Chen et al., 2013;). While these publications address a variety of organisational or contextual issues, a consistent finding has been that even though healthcare professionals demonstrate a positive attitude towards research, there exists a lack of confidence in their research knowledge and in their ability to appraise research reports (Gerrish et al., 2008; Lyons et al.; 2011).

In the process of translating research findings into practice, a key step is determining if those findings *should* be implemented. This is no easy task given that contemporary healthcare is highly-pressured, complex and resource restricted. Moreover, technological advances and the explosion of available knowledge mean that the sheer volume of available research on a vast array of topics is itself a barrier to translation to practice. Even searching and locating appropriate research is a highly skilled activity. In addition, research with its ever expanding range of methodologies and methods is becoming increasingly complex. Yet, we would argue that this increasing complexity and unlimited access to research makes the ability to analyse and interpret research even more important for deciding best practice in any given situation. In order to do this healthcare practitioners must understand and have knowledge of research and the research process and possess the skills to make judgements about its quality and the significance of its findings for practice. Becoming research aware is the first step in developing the skills to make these judgements.

Becoming Research Aware

In our modern world, it could be said that the majority of people have some level of awareness of healthcare research. This is because most weeks there are reports in the popular media about the findings of studies related to disease processes, treatments, and therapies that are deemed to be of interest to the general public. Some topics are considered more newsworthy than others because of their perceived importance to the health of society but they represent only a fraction of the research studies that are being conducted in healthcare. For example, if the findings of a research study point to actual or possible developments in the treatment of cancer, it is likely that it will receive considerable attention. A key point, however, is that reports in the media are just that and they tend to focus on the results of the study rather than if the study was well conducted and therefore if the results are credible. Thus, there is a distinct difference between awareness of the results of studies and being research aware as a practitioner of healthcare. As indicated above, healthcare practitioners must not only be aware of the research that is being conducted within their field of interest but must also possess the skills to make judgements about the quality of that research. This is not easy and considerable effort is needed to develop research literacy.

However, when students of healthcare are introduced to research in their undergraduate programmes many find it difficult to see what it has to do with practice. Sometimes practitioners and students are fearful of research and do not understand the terminology. Doing research can be seen as an elitist activity and at times the manner in which it is presented in academic journals perpetuates this perception.

Yet, research awareness does not necessarily mean undertaking the research yourself but it does mean being able to analyse the components of various research studies in order to determine what is good research and therefore what has most applicability for our patients. To do this, we must develop an understanding of the research process and what is required at each stage. This includes being cognisant of the language of research, the methodologies, research designs, methods of data collection and data analysis, determinants of quality, ethical issues and factors related to dissemination and application or implementation of the findings. This is important because research is not determined as being 'good' simply by virtue of its focus. There are potentially innumerable topics in healthcare research that are worthy of study. However, it is the manner in which the question is posed and how well the methodologies and methods that are employed to undertake it that determines ultimately if it is good research (Ellis, 2010).

Knowing how to appraise research reports is a significant precursor to research utilisation, which is defined by Estabrooks (1999a) as the transformation of findings into interventions that can be used in practice. Studies have measured and confirmed three forms of research utilisation (conceptual, instrumental and persuasive) among nurses (Estabrooks, 1999a, 1999b; Profetto-McGrath et al., 2003; Kenny, 2005; Milner et al., 2005; Forsman et al., 2009; Wangensteen et al., 2011). Conceptual research utilisation refers to changes of opinion or changes in how the nurse thinks about a particular clinical situation because of research although it may not result in a direct change in action. Instrumental (direct) research utilisation is about the concrete application of research findings such as in practice or policy guidelines. Finally, persuasive research utilisation refers to the use of research to persuade others, usually those who make decisions, to make changes to policies, practices or conditions pertaining to nurses, patients and/or the health of individuals or groups (Estabrooks, 1999a). Conceptual and instrumental research utilisation are used more often among nurses than persuasive research utilisation.

These studies have found, however, that overall research utilisation among qualified nurses is low despite the emphasis on appraisal and use of research evidence in undergraduate study. Furthermore, Forsman et al. (2009) found a decrease in research utilisation among practitioners who were three years post-graduation compared with those who were one year post-graduation. While these studies do not focus on organisational or situational factors such as environment, resources and time (Gerrish et al., 2008) that facilitate or hamper research utilisation, they do identify individual determinants. These factors are seen to be of considerable importance and include knowledge of and attitude towards research utilisation, as well as critical thinking skills such as being open-minded, inquisitive and systematic. The greater the number of practitioners who have a strong individual commitment to research utilisation the more likely it may be that a supportive environment for research utilisation will emerge.

Thus, becoming research aware is the beginning of a long-term commitment to research utilisation for the ultimate benefit of those for whom we care. While we can never know all there is to know about research or even the focus of that research we can contribute to creating healthcare environments that enable practitioners to utilise research evidence.

Chapter Summary

This introductory chapter has provided the historical context for the subsequent chapters of this book. Research was defined as being concerned with scrutinising an issue of interest using a structured method for the purpose of refinement, validation or refutation of current knowledge and/or the creation of new knowledge. The focus of research as the development of propositional knowledge was outlined within the context of the branch of philosophy known as epistemology. The relationships between research and knowledge, research and theory and research and practice were outlined and incorporated consideration of issues such as the influence of epistemology on the development of knowledge and the impact of philosophical thinking on approaches to theory development. The importance of scientific evidence from research as one element of evidence-based practice was presented with other essential elements being identified as individual clinical expertise and the needs of the individual patient. The chapter concluded by exploring the importance of becoming research aware, the skills needed to be research aware and how this is related to research utilisation in practice.

Key Points

- Contemporary research is concerned with examining or scrutinising an issue of interest which may lead to refinement, validation or refutation of current knowledge and/or the creation of new knowledge.
- Research is referred to as empirical research and is synonymous with the conscious application of a structured method.
- There are different types of knowledge that can be broadly classified into propositional, procedural and personal knowledge.
- The focus of research is the development of propositional knowledge.
- There are two opposing philosophical traditions known as rationalism and empiricism. These have resulted in inductive (bottom-up) and deductive (top-down) approaches to undertaking research.
- The ultimate aim of all scientific research is to devise theories that describe, explain, predict or control aspects of the world.
- Knowledge generated from research is one form of evidence.
- Scientific evidence, clinical expertise and the needs of the individual patient comprise evidence-based practice (EBP).
- Research awareness means being able to analyse the components of various research studies.

Useful Online Resources

www.socialresearchmethods.net/kb/dedind.php
www.medicine.ox.ac.uk/bandolier/

2

The Research Process at a Glance

Introduction

The terms research and the research process often invoke feelings of apprehension and dread in novice researchers and students. The language and terminology encountered when reading a research article or hearing research discussed often seem alien, and the research process can seem confusing to those who are unfamiliar with its structure. However, well conducted research follows a well-defined sequence of steps and these steps are what have become known as the research process.

Undertaking a research study is similar to undertaking a journey and like any journey it has a point of origin, a planned route and a final destination. If you are unsure where you are starting, the route to your destination can be tortuous. Using the same analogy, if you do not know where you are going, or how you will get there, you could end up anywhere. When undertaking research, the research process acts like a route map that guides the researcher towards a robust outcome. The process identifies the steps, but it is up to the researcher to adhere to the process. The research problem is the point of origin, developing a research question or hypothesis identifies what you are attempting to achieve, that is, your destination. Finally, when you reach your destination you will want to share your knowledge and experiences of the journey with others. The other steps resemble points of reference along the way that help to keep you on the correct route. Knowledge of the process can thus alert a reader that a study may have strayed from the steps, and that the robustness of the study may be in question.

Understanding the research process is important for those who plan to read or use research-based evidence as part of their work, as it is the first step in critically appraising a research study and being able to identify the strengths and limitations therein. Application of the process is important for those either preparing a research proposal or undertaking research as adherence to the process will increase the likelihood that the proposal or study will be robust. The purpose of this chapter is to give the reader an overview of the research process and to introduce the steps in the process.

☑ Learning Outcomes ☑

By the end of this chapter you should be able to:

- Recognise the research process
- List the steps in the research process
- Briefly outline the purpose of each step of the research process

---

The Research Process

The research process can be described as a relatively linear series of steps that can guide the researcher from the start of a study (identifying a research problem), to the conclusion (discovering an answer) (Polit & Beck, 2014). The steps have a logical progression and generally occur in the order described in the box below. There can be some minor variations in this sequence between quantitative research, qualitative research and a systematic review. These variations will be discussed in relation to the individual steps. The steps in the process can be categorised into groups of related activities (see the box below).

Steps in the Research Process

Developing a Researchable Topic

- Identifying the Research Problem / Topic of Interest
- Reviewing the Literature
- Devising a Research Question / Hypothesis

Organising your Research

- Selecting a methodology
- Identifying the population and selecting a sample
- Planning the method of data collection
- Respecting ethical principles
- Demonstrating rigour/trustworthiness

Gathering and analysing information

- Gathering data
- Analysing data
- Discussing and interpreting the results and implications for practice
- Disseminating the results

Developing a Researchable Topic

The first step that a researcher must achieve when developing a topic to research is to identify the purpose of the study. In this there are a number of items that need to be considered. If the research to be undertaken is an assignment for a course, there may be a timeframe in which it must be completed and a word limit that will restrict how much can be written. With these in mind it is important to select a project that is achievable, not only from an assignment perspective but also from a research perspective. Not all questions are researchable, for example 'Is there a God?' While many people will perhaps have strong beliefs on this topic, it is not possible to gather empirical evidence to either refute or support an answer to this question. So from this perspective the research problem or topic of interest must be one that is researchable. As can be seen from the previous box (p. 13) there are three steps involved in developing a researchable topic. The first step is to identify a research problem or topic of interest.

Identifying a Research Problem / Topic of Interest / Broad Question

The first step in the research process is identifying a problem that needs to be investigated. While this may seem a simple step, it is probably one of the most important decisions a researcher will make when undertaking a study. If the research problem is interesting and achievable, it can help keep a researcher on the journey through the research process. Alternatively, a research problem that is poorly devised can leave a researcher feeling swamped and unable to cope (Coughlan et al., 2013). How to identify a research problem is discussed in detail in Chapter 3.

Reviewing the Literature

Once the research problem or topic of interest has been identified the next step is to search the literature for information related to the topic. Among other things, reviewing the literature can help the researcher become familiar with the current state of knowledge on the topic, identify if there are gaps in the literature and to develop or refine a research question (Cronin et al., 2008). In reviewing the literature, the researcher critically appraises the studies included and highlights the strengths and limitations of these for the reader.

With some qualitative methodologies there is variation in respect of when the literature review is undertaken. For example, in grounded theory, the literature review may be undertaken after the data has been collected and analysed. This approach is taken so the researcher will not be influenced by the literature when collecting the data (Streubert & Carpenter, 2011). A more in-depth discussion in relation to reviewing the literature can be found in Chapter 4.

Devising a Research Question / Hypothesis

Information gleaned from the literature review is used to formulate an interrogative (questioning) statement that clearly identifies what the researcher is seeking from the research. The research question helps identify the most appropriate methodology for the study, and as such, becomes a link between the original research problem and the research design (Grove et al., 2013).

Normally the formulation of a research question occurs after the literature has been searched and analysed. However, in the case of a Systematic Review, a very clear and specific research question is required before the review can be undertaken. This is because a Systematic Review is considered a form of research in itself and an unambiguous research question is required in order to have a clear indication of what literature needs to be included in the review (Coughlan et al., 2013).

A hypothesis is similar to a research question but without the interrogative. It is a statement that clearly identifies what the researcher is seeking to demonstrate through research. Hypotheses are used in experimental and quasi-experimental research and in some correlational studies. Research questions and hypotheses are discussed in detail in Chapter 3.

Organising Your Research

Once researchers have an idea of where they are going with their research the next consideration is determining how they are going to get there, that is, how it will be undertaken. The next series of steps deal with the issues of identifying the appropriate methodology, selecting participants, planning how the necessary data will be collected, ensuring that this method of data gathering is trustworthy and that the rights of the participants are protected.

Selecting a Methodology

The first step in organising a research study is to identify a research methodology. The methodology selected should be the best one to answer the research question. There are a number of approaches to undertaking research but these have been classified broadly as quantitative (studies that collect numerical data) and qualitative (studies that collect narrative or words). Quantitatively-based studies are commonly associated with the positivist and post-positivist paradigms while those that are qualitatively based tend to be aligned with interpretive/constructivist and critical/advocacy paradigms. See Chapter 5 for a discussion of paradigms.

Quantitatively-based research is interested in measurable outcomes. Opinion polls are one example where, for instance, satisfaction with political parties is measured. However, rather than focusing on proof, post-positivist researchers are interested in probabilities. For example, how probable is it that cigarette smoking leads to the development of lung cancer? In other words, can an association between the variable 'cigarette smoking' and the variable 'lung cancer' be demonstrated? In seeking to demonstrate this association, the researcher has hypothesised that a potential link exists and is therefore testing this belief.

Qualitatively-based research on the other hand is interested in describing or understanding phenomenon rather than measuring or counting the incidence of exposure. Consequently outcomes lead to theory development.

There are strengths and limitations to quantitatively- and qualitatively-based research methodologies. Mixed methods is an approach that uses both the aforementioned methodologies in order to maximise the strengths and reduce the limitations of the individual approaches. Explanatory designs use a qualitative approach to develop a greater understanding of the quantitative data, and exploratory designs can use a quantitative approach, for example to test a theory that emerges from the qualitative data (Grove et al., 2013). Advocacy or Emancipatory approaches regard research as means of highlighting social problems and inequities within society, and bringing about change (Polit & Beck, 2014).

Once a methodology is selected then a research method can be identified. Although often discussed as being synonymous, methodologies and methods are different. Methodologies offer a broader, philosophical overview of research which can be further subdivided into approaches that describe how the research should be undertaken. This description of how the research should be undertaken is the method. An overview of some of the approaches associated with the two main paradigms can be seen in the box below.

Paradigms and Associated Methodologies

Positivist/Post-positivist Paradigm

- Quantitative Descriptive research e.g. survey
- Comparative descriptive research
- Correlational Research
- Quasi-experimental research
- Experimental research

Interpretivist/Constructivist Paradigm

- Qualitative Descriptive Research
- Phenomenology
- Grounded Theory
- Ethnography

Advocacy (Emancipatory) Approaches

- Participatory Action Research

In selecting the methodology and the method, the researcher is expected to justify why they were selected. This includes recognition of philosophical theory that underpins the approach and thus an acknowledgement of how the research will be conducted. Research methodologies are considered in more detail in Chapter 5.

Identifying the Population and Selecting a Sample

When undertaking research it is important to know the population of interest. A population in research are all the individuals who could potentially participate in the research and to whom the results will apply. Usually, populations apply to large numbers of individuals who cannot all be included in the research study. Therefore, a sample of the population is used.

In research that collects numerical data, the sample should ideally be representative of the population, that is, as close to a miniature version of the population as possible. The purpose of this is to try to generalise the results of the study back to the population. The type of sampling method used to achieve this is called probability sampling. When using probability sampling the larger the sample the more likely it is to be representative. As a result researchers collecting numerical data tend to use large samples (Grove et al., 2013).

Conversely, in research that collects narrative (words) the purpose is to identify individuals' experiences of the phenomenon being studied, so samples do not need to be as large as in studies that collect numerical data. Consequently, it is important that the individuals selected to participate in the study have experience of the phenomenon of interest. This type of sampling is known as purposive sampling. Ideally, the endpoint for sample selection in qualitatively-based research is when 'data saturation' has been achieved. Data saturation implies that no new information is being gleaned from participants about the phenomenon of interest (Streubert & Carpenter, 2011). However, in the practice of conducting research, data saturation remains an aspiration and is rarely achieved. Although some might consider this a limitation, it does not mean the study data is inaccurate. It means, simply, that there may be other experiences in the target population that have not been recorded in the study. Sampling and sample selecting will be further discussed in Chapter 6.

Planning the Method of Data Collection

The next step in the process is deciding how the data will be collected. To some degree this will have been determined by the methodology that was selected. For instance, in experimental, quasi-experimental or non-experimental studies that collect numerical data, researchers may be attempting to find patterns or results that can be generalised to the whole population and therefore in-depth interviews or focus groups would not be suitable approaches to data collection. Thus, in survey research the most popular method of data gathering is postal questionnaire as it can be administered to a large sample quickly and efficiently with minimal cost.

Conversely, if researchers are using methodologies that are gathering narrative (words) they will be more interested in the individual experiences of the participants and therefore would not use experiments or questionnaires as data gathering methods. In research that collects narrative (words) one of the most common methods of data collection is interview. Interviews can be semi-structured or unstructured (Ryan et al., 2009). Overall, what is important is that the approach to data collection is congruent with the research approach adopted. The methods of data collection will be further developed and discussed in Chapter 9.

Respecting Ethical Principles

Evidence from history demonstrates that without strong ethical principles being adhered to, there is a risk that the rights of individuals may not always be preserved.

Studies undertaken in the name of research have been seen to deprive individuals of the right to informed consent and even withheld viable treatments so that the progression of disease might be studied (Tuskegee Syphilis Study 1932–1972) (Tuskegee University, 2013); to infect children with intellectual disabilities to study the natural progression of a disease (Willowbrook Study) (Rothman, 1982); and to inject cancer cells into elderly patients to see if people without cancer responded differently when exposed to cancer than those who had developed the disease naturally (Jewish Chronic Disease Hospital Study) (Katz, 1972). These and other such cases led to the development of ethical codes and guidelines that enshrine the rights of all individuals and usually entail special considerations for vulnerable groups. Included in these guidelines are the right of the individual to autonomy, beneficence, non-maleficence and justice (Beauchamp & Childress, 2013).

Hospitals and other institutions that are responsible for individuals usually have ethical committees that will review any research proposals to ensure that all ethical principles are adhered to, before deciding whether to give permission to undertake a study. Third level colleges will usually undertake a similar process before giving students permission to proceed with a research study. Ultimately however, it is the responsibility of the researcher to ensure that the proposed study is ethically robust and protects the rights of the participants. Health and Social Care research in the UK is governed by the National Research Ethics Service (NRES). This group offers guidelines as to whether ethical approval is required for a research study (www.hra-decisiontools.org.uk/ethics/index.html) and online application forms (https://www.myresearchproject.org.uk/). Further information on ethics in research can be found in Chapter 7.

Demonstrating Rigour / Trustworthiness

When undertaking a research study, it is important to ensure that the results will be trustworthy. In research that collects numerical data, validity and reliability are used to demonstrate thoroughness and robustness. Validity can be external or internal. External validity refers to whether the findings of the study can be generalised. One of the criteria in this regard is the representativeness of the sample. Internal validity examines the data gathering instrument to determine if it measures what it is supposed to measure. Reliability is the degree of consistency the research instrument has when recording data on the phenomenon being studied. When testing reliability there are a number of facets that need to be considered including stability, internal consistency and equivalence. An overview of validity and reliability can be seen in Table 2.1.

In a range of qualitative research designs, the concepts of validity and reliability are not always congruent with the underlying methodological philosophies (Grove et al., 2013) thus other means of ensuring trustworthiness were devised. In qualitative research rigour is interested in the trustworthiness of the results. Lincoln and Guba (1985) identified the criteria of credibility, dependability, transferability, confirmability and authenticity as the means of demonstrating rigour. A brief summary of these criteria is presented in Table 2.1.

Table 2.1   An overview of the validity, reliability and rigour

Quantitatively-Based Research – Validity

External Validity	Concerned with the generalisability of the findings
Internal Validity	
• Face Validity	Face validity is concerned with reading the study instrument and judging whether the questions 'appear' to measure what they are supposed to
• Content validity	Content validity considers if the content of the data collection instrument is inclusive and applicable to the research question
• Criterion-related validity (concurrent and predictive)	Criterion validity is used to compare one data gathering instrument or method with another. If data from the two methods can be compared in tandem and have similar results the instrument is deemed to have concurrent validity
	If the instrument can accurately identify how an individual will respond or behave in a particular situation it can be said to have predictive validity (for example an entrance examination that attempts to select students that will be more suited to a course)
• Construct Validity	Construct validity attempts to ensure that there is a congruity between the variables of the conceptual frameworks and how the researcher plans to measure these. This can be a difficult concept to test

Quantitatively-Based Research – Reliability

Stability	The stability of an instrument refers to the degree to which it generates similar findings from the same group on different occasions
Internal Consistency	Internal consistency is used to determine the degree to which items on a questionnaire measure a particular variable. Items with a strong internal consistency are said to be homogeneous
Equivalence	The most common use of equivalence in clinical research is inter-rater reliability in observational studies, where both observers need to be measuring their observations similarly

Qualitatively-Based Research – Rigour

Credibility	Credibility attempts to demonstrate that the findings and interpretations accurately describe the participants' experiences
Dependability	This criterion attempts to determine how sound the findings are. Credibility is an essential component of this criterion as without credibility there can be no dependability (Streubert & Carpenter, 2011)
Transferability	If the researcher can show that the findings of a study are applicable to other groups or in other settings, the study is said to have transferability
Confirmability	The criterion of confirmability is achieved by the researcher leaving a clear audit trail as to how the data and evidence were managed and how conclusions were derived (Streubert & Carpenter, 2011)
Authenticity	To establish authenticity, a researcher needs to be able to re-create the reality experienced by individual participants, so as to allow the reader a deeper understanding of the theme being described (Polit & Beck, 2014)

(see Chapter 8 for additional detail)

Gathering and Analysing Information

The next stage is concerned with achieving the outcome of the research study. The steps involve gathering information about the phenomenon or topic of interest, analysing that data and arriving at an outcome. The last step involves putting the findings in context and clarifying for the reader what the results mean in the relation to practice.

Gathering Data

As stated earlier the process of data collection will be determined by the methodology chosen and the question the research study poses. Experimental, quasi-experimental and non-experimental studies generally collect a numerical form of data. This data is collected in its entirety before being analysed. In studies that collect narrative data and which focus on capturing the individual's experience of the phenomenon, analysis can occur concurrently with data collection.

Prior to commencing data collection, a pilot study or pilot interview is often undertaken. A pilot study or interview uses the same methods to select participants and collect data as are proposed for the main study. It can be helpful as potential problems that can occur during data collection can be identified and strategies to manage these can be developed (Grove et al., 2013). Generally, data gathered and participants involved in the pilot study or pilot interview are excluded from the main study.

Analysing Data

Data gathered in a research study needs to be presented to the reader in a format that is clear and succinct. The organisation of this information to formulate the findings of the study is called data analysis. In experimental, quasi-experimental and non-experimental research that collects numerical data, statistical analysis is undertaken. There are two types of statistical analysis – descriptive and inferential. Descriptive statistics literally describe the participants by their demographic details and the pattern of their responses, for example, how many participants in each specific age group responded in a particular way. Descriptive quantitative studies only use descriptive statistics. However, descriptive statistics are always included in studies undertaking inferential statistics. Inferential statistics are used to determine the likelihood that the results of the study occurred by chance, or if they are a true reflection of the population – in other words can inferences be made to the target population?

In many qualitative research studies, the researcher is concerned with data in the form of words and text as opposed to the numerical data. The researcher is expected to become very familiar with the data so much so that the term 'immersed in the data' is used. Once familiar with the data the researcher attempts to code it and reduce it down to a number of themes that represent the key concepts that recur within the data. There are a number of different instruments for analysing qualitative data, some of which are specific to particular methodological approaches. Further information on analysing data is presented in Chapter 10.

Discussing and Interpreting the Results and the Implications for Practice

In the discussion section the researcher links the findings back to the research question, and considers the meaning and implications of the results. In doing this the quantitative researcher will discuss the findings with regard to the studies presented in the literature review; while the qualitative researcher will search for literature to support the discoveries made in the study. Interpretation of the results includes not only the findings but also an analysis of how the study itself was undertaken, as both strengths and limitations will impact on any inferences made. No research study is perfect, however it is better for the researcher to recognise and identify the limitations and strengths in his/her own study. As the limitations are discussed the researcher has the opportunity to deliberate on perhaps the inevitability of some limitations and suggest ways that others might be avoided in the future.

The discussion section usually concludes with recommendations and implications for practice. These are usually presented in the form of suggestions as to how practice may be improved as a result of implementing the findings of the study, or how further research would be prudent before implementing change (Grove et al., 2013). Suggestions for future related research can also be included here. It is important to remember throughout this section that results, interpretations and implications are tentative and should be written in a format that suggests that these outcomes are what the results appear to be indicating, rather than absolute fact (Polit & Beck, 2012).

Disseminating the Results

Undertaking a research study is an empty task if the results are not made available so that others may learn from and build on this information. It is therefore important that this data is shared with peers and other interested groups. There are a number of different ways in which this information can be disseminated and this will be discussed in Chapter 11.

Chapter Summary

Undertaking a piece of research is similar to undertaking a new journey. It is important to know where you are starting from and where you are going to. The research process acts as a road map that guides the researcher through the research journey. For the novice researcher familiarity with the research process is a fundamental requirement whether you are reading research, preparing a research proposal or planning to undertake a piece of research. A knowledge and understanding of the process will help the individual reading research to critically appraise a study and identify its strengths and limitations. For individuals preparing a research proposal or planning to do research, an understanding of, and adherence to the process will increase the likelihood that the proposal or study will be robust.

🔑 Key Points 🔑

- The research process is a series of steps that can guide a novice researcher when reading a piece of research.
- Poor adherence to the steps of the research process can undermine the robustness of the study.
- Knowledge of the research process can be helpful when critically analysing the methodological rigour of a piece of research.

3

What are Research Problems, Questions, Hypotheses, Aims and Objectives?

Introduction

At a multidisciplinary clinical team meeting, early one Thursday morning, a staff midwife asked the question; *'why do we listen continuously to the baby's heart rate* [by a machine called the electronic fetal monitor] *during labour when we know that there are no research studies that support this in low risk, healthy pregnant women?'*

The question was initially posed out of simple curiosity based on the midwife's observations during her daily clinical practice and through her awareness of non-compliance with the local policy guidelines. It soon became apparent that this was an important clinical question that required a clear answer. The problem lay within the midwife's question; that is, midwives were listening to the baby's heart beat continuously during labour in low risk healthy women. An electronic machine that picks up the baby's heart rate via an ultrasound disc attached to a woman's abdomen was being used for this purpose. Current evidence, however, does not support this practice in low risk pregnant women. The research question arises from this problem; why was this still being done? The foundations of a clinically important research study had been laid.

The focus of this chapter is to explore how you might come to identify research problems, questions and hypotheses. Determining whether a research question is actually researchable or not, will be discussed. Differentiating between a research question and a research hypothesis will be addressed. Finally, setting research aims and objectives so that a research question might be effectively answered, will be explored.

☑ **Learning Outcomes** ☑

By the end of this Chapter you should be able to:

- Identify sources for research topics
- Understand the term 'research problem'
- Understand the term 'research question'
- Formulate a research question
- Differentiate between a research question and a research hypothesis
- Understand the terms research aims and objectives.

The Research Topic

All research work must begin by identifying a topic of interest or a general subject area for study. Although this might appear to be stating the obvious, without having a clear research topic any plans for a subsequent study will have no foundation from which to develop. For some, pinning down a broad topic of interest can be difficult and challenging. For others, it may be fairly straightforward as it might be an area of healthcare that they have been interested in for some time. Alternatively, a topic may already have been identified by a funding agency and a researcher is commissioned to conduct the study. Whatever the case, choosing a subject area for study enables a researcher to determine what it is they want to study and why. It also provides future directions for the study as it is from the chosen topic of interest that specific research problems and questions will arise. When reading published research papers, in the main, you will find the source of the research topic and the rationale for conducting the study in the introductory section. Alternatively, the acknowledgements section, at the end of a paper, might provide information on a funding source. This could indicate that the research study was commissioned by a particular funding body.

Numerous sources abound within healthcare from which research topics can arise. A researcher, depending on where their particular interests lie, might draw on one or several of these sources. Here are some common sources that can be considered:

Clinical Practice

Clinical practice provides a rich source of topics for study and is likely the most commonly drawn-upon source. Topics continuously emerge during our daily practice and/or our encounters with people, clients, colleagues and other healthcare professionals. A topic might emerge from a personal interest in a specific area of clinical healthcare. Alternatively, it may emerge from observations of variations in healthcare practices, either within healthcare units or between units. A good example of this was evidence of variations in practice in routine episiotomy (a small cut to the perineum as a baby is being born) which varied from 14 per cent to 96 per cent across maternity units in the United Kingdom. This prompted the conduct of an important research study that evaluated the use of routine versus selective episiotomy in first time labouring women (Sleep et al., 1984). The results of this study provided a lack of evidence for routine episiotomy. Consequently, clinical practice has changed whereby routine episiotomy is rarely ever now performed with selective episiotomy the current norm.

Education/Classroom Discussions

Classroom discussions often provide undergraduate healthcare students with topics for research study. This is because it is during these discussions that differences between what the theoretical foundations suggest and what actually happens in clinical practice can arise. The classroom environment can provide the opportunity to reflect on these and to discuss with colleagues why such variations might exist. In this sense, a thought process, which could ultimately lead to the development of a research study, might begin.

As an activity, consider some classroom discussions that you recently have been involved in. Did any disparities between theory and clinical practice arise? If yes, consider if any of these might form the basis of a broad topic of interest for study.

ACTIVITY 3.1

Reviewing the Literature

Reviewing healthcare literature can provide important areas for research study. As can often be the case, rather than actually seeking topics for study, a research topic can unexpectedly emerge from reading the literature. For instance, we might find ourselves reading research papers in an area of healthcare simply out of interest or perhaps for purposes of advancing our knowledge in the area. This might reveal a lack of evidence related to some (or all) aspects of the topic. In this sense, a review of the literature can identify a gap in the evidence-base that could provide topics that warrant further study. Specific recommendations that might be provided in the literature can also provide topics for research study. A good example of this appears in a systematic review on the topic of physiotherapy after traumatic brain injury (Hellweg & Johannes, 2008). This review concluded that some recommendations for the effectiveness of physical therapy interventions could be made. However, the authors go on to say that there are many questions concerning the treatment of humans with traumatic brain injury which have not been investigated so far. This type of finding might encourage an individual with a particular interest in this area to develop and conduct a research study to evaluate treatments that have not been investigated thus far so that a greater body of evidence on this topic might be established.

Health Service Users (Including Consumer Group Associations)

Concerns raised by consumer groups and health service users often provide important sources for research topics. An example of this can be seen in the Deloitte

Centre for Health Solutions annual survey (Deloitte, 2012). Deloitte, since 2008, have annually surveyed U.S. adults to gauge their opinions and expectations about the healthcare system. For example, the surveys focus on issues such as the use of the system, performance of the system, unmet needs and health reform. The results from these surveys can identify areas of consumer dissatisfaction, satisfaction and/ or need. These various findings, in turn, could prompt a researcher to examine any particular issue further to determine how service users' needs might best be met.

Society

Societal concerns often identify important areas for research work. These concerns may arise at national or international level. For example, concerns expressed by particular groups in a society, such as those suffering from particular conditions, might prompt investigations into the specific healthcare needs of these groups. Alternatively, global health concerns, such as outbreaks of particular types of infections or diseases (consider the AIDS pandemic or, more recently, the global concerns resulting from the avian and swine flu outbreaks) might prompt healthcare researchers to conduct research to explore these issues from an international perspective. The World Health Organization is an example of one such organisation that conducts research studies arising from issues of global healthcare concern.

As you can see, there are many sources from which research topics can arise. Irrespective of the source, however, it is essential that a researcher is also interested in the chosen topic. This is because undertaking any type of research involves immersing oneself deeply in the subject area. There is the potential for some researchers to engage with a subject area simply because it is accessible and available to them. A lack of interest in a topic can have detrimental effects on both the researcher and on the research study. It may lead to a negative experience for the researcher. It may discourage a researcher from engaging with future research projects. It may result in lack-lustre efforts by the researcher which can compromise the integrity and rigour (accuracy or thoroughness) of the research process. It also has the potential to result in the research study being abandoned. Abandoning a study following commencement has numerous consequences, not least of all, a derogation of ethical obligations to complete the study and a failed obligation to the study participants and/or to the potential healthcare benefits that the study might bring.

ACTIVITY 3.2

To get you thinking about topics for research, list three broad subject areas for study. Identify the source of these topics. Write down why they are of interest to you.

Once a broad topic of interest has been identified, the next step is to identify the problem associated with that topic. Throughout the remainder of this chapter broad healthcare topics will be drawn upon to exemplify the subsequent steps of identifying the research problem, defining the research question and setting research aims and objectives.

The Research Problem

A research problem, often referred to as a 'problem statement', can be described as an aspect of a topic that might be troubling, concerning or thought provoking and perplexing. It does not necessarily indicate that there is 'a problem' in the commonly understood sense (that is, something 'bad' or 'difficult'). Rather it may simply be some concern over a deficit in knowledge related to a particular topic. Alternatively, it may be an issue that arises during discussions with clinical colleagues that causes uncertainty or confusion. A good example of this is when healthcare professionals have differing opinions on how something might best be done. Finally, it may be an element of a topic for which a researcher personally knows little about and wishes to find out more. Whatever the origin of the research problem, the essential factor is that a research problem is something that needs to be solved. It is through the conduct of research that this is achieved.

As with the research topic, it is important that a researcher allows some time to consider the problem(s) associated with a topic. One activity that can be performed to assist with this is to conduct a brainstorming exercise whereby all of the associated issues are written down and explored. Possible problems associated with each of the various issues might then be highlighted. Figure 3.1 provides an example of a brainstorming exercise on the topic of preterm birth. Table 3.1 provides problem statements associated with each of the identified issues. Importantly, as you will see from the example, a research problem is always declarative and not interrogative. What this means, is that a research problem is always written as a statement or 'declared', hence the term 'problem statement', and it is not posed in a question format. It is from the research problem/problem statement that the research question will arise and be asked.

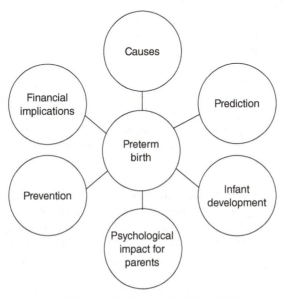

Figure 3.1   Brainstorming exercise on the topic of preterm birth

Table 3.1　Developing problem statements

Topic	Associated Issues	Problem Statement
Preterm Birth	Causes	Infection causes preterm birth
	Prediction	Preterm birth might be predicted if we monitor, more closely, women who are at a higher risk of preterm birth
	Infant development	Babies who are born preterm are at a higher risk of developing neurological long-term deficits
	Psychological impact	Preterm birth impacts on the psychological wellbeing of parents
	Prevention	Targeted interventions might prevent preterm birth
	Financial implications	The resource demands associated with preterm birth negatively affect the healthcare service provider

As is evident from Table 3.1, there is the potential for a number of problem statements to arise from one broad topic. It would be impossible for a single research study to solve all of these problems; rather a number of very different types of studies would be required to effectively do this. The challenge for a researcher is to determine which problem statement should be subjected to study. In some instances this choice might be based on a researcher's particular preference. Alternatively, it may be a problem area already commissioned for study. Either way, when clarifying a research problem for purposes of study, an effective researcher will initially enter into a process of consideration, deliberation, questioning and discussion on all of the problem statements. Consulting clinical colleagues, other healthcare researchers, experts in the field and/or the literature might also be helpful when attempting to narrow down a problem statement for purposes of study. Ultimately, when clarifying a research problem, it is essential that the problem bears relevance to clinical practice and/or is likely to contribute to the theoretical advancement of the subject area.

It is worth noting, at this point, that problem statements are seldom presented as distinct statements in the text of published journals papers. Rather, the problem statement is usually embedded within the background or introduction section of a paper. Below is an excerpt from the introductory paragraph of a maternity care research report. The problem statement is embedded within this paragraph. See if you can identify it.

> Pervading perceptions of what constitutes a pregnancy-related risk differs between and within groups including medical experts, midwives, and childbearing women … and there is a lack of understanding and clarity on what constitutes 'risk' in maternity care. As such, the concept of risk in maternity care warrants an in-depth exploration and analysis. (Smith et al., 2012: 126)

The topic of interest can be identified here as 'risk in maternity care'. Identifying the problem statement, however, might not be as clear. Returning to the definition of a problem statement we can remind ourselves that it is something that must be solved. With this in mind, the problem statement in the above example could be considered and re-written as: *'there are differing perceptions of pregnancy-related risk and there is a lack of understanding and clarity on what constitutes risk in maternity care.'* Based on this declaration the researchers must solve this problem by developing a study which will provide greater understanding and clarity on risk in maternity care.

3.1   Thoughts and Tips

As a tip in becoming familiar with identifying problem statements, have a highlighter pen to hand when reading research papers (or use the highlighter function if reading papers in electronic form). Highlight what you think might be the research problem. If necessary or appropriate re-write this as a distinct problem statement. Share this with your colleagues to see if they agree or disagree with your decision.

Formulating the Research Question

Once the research problem has been clarified, the next step for a researcher is to pose a specific, clearly defined research question. A research question could be thought of as a conversion of the problem statement into a question format that will be answered through the conduct of a study. Defining a research question is a fundamental aspect of a research study as it informs the future direction of the study. For example, a clear research question will guide the design of the study, where the study will take place, who will take part in the study and what information should be obtained during the study. Without a clearly defined research question the choice of study design may be inappropriate, the quality of the study may be compromised and the results of the study may have little meaning. Therefore, as with the research problem, it is imperative that a researcher spends some time developing and formulating their research question. To assist in the initial stages of this, a researcher could ask some basic questions related to the problem as follows;

- What do I see and do in clinical practice?
- What does the literature say?
- Are there discrepancies between what I see and do and what I know or what the literature says?
- Is this the best way to do this/is there another way to do this?
- What do others think?
- What are the elements of this problem that could be improved?

The answer to these questions might help in developing a broad research question. After further thought the broad research question will be narrowed down to a specific, clearly defined question for purposes of study.

Formulating a research question is best achieved by following a step-by-step process. Here are some useful steps that a researcher could follow:

1. Identify the broad topic of interest
2. Identify the research problem and write down the problem statement
3. Describe a broad research question that will solve the research problem or address the problem statement
4. Review the relevant literature
5. Clearly define/refine the research question for purposes of study

Provided in the box below is a worked example of using this process to formulate a research question on the topic of preterm birth.

Formulating the Research Question

1. Topic of interest: Preterm birth.
2. Research problem/problem statement: Infection is the cause of preterm birth in 20 per cent–40 per cent of cases.
3. Broad research question: If infection in pregnancy is prevented and/or treated early will this prevent preterm birth in some women?
4. Review of the literature: Antibiotics treat infection. The use of prophylactic antibiotics in women at risk of preterm birth may have the potential to prevent preterm birth resulting from infectious causes.
5. Define/refine the research question: Does prophylactic antibiotic therapy prevent preterm birth in women who are at a higher risk of preterm birth?

Note how the broad research question is further narrowed and refined to provide a question that is purposively directive for the study. So, based on the above research question, the researcher must now conduct a study that will examine whether antibiotic therapy is effective, women who are at a higher risk of having a preterm birth must be accessed and the study must take place in a setting where pregnant women are available.

Reviewing the literature is a very important step prior to formulating a final research question. There are a number of reasons for this such as establishing what is already known about the topic of interest and/or identifying gaps in the literature. More importantly, however, a review of the literature must be undertaken to establish that the research question has not already been answered. Research studies can be resource consuming. It would be a waste of time and money to conduct a study that provides evidence on a topic when there is ample evidence already available. An example of this can be illustrated in a discussion piece provided by Paterson (2001). In the discussion a nurse queries why intravenous (IV) tubing in the intensive care unit should be changed every 48 hours rather than every 72 hours. Conducting a study to determine whether every 48 hours is better than every 72 hours is not appropriate here as there is sufficient evidence from previous studies to demonstrate that 48 hours is preferable. In reality, however, in the clinical setting, IV tubing is often changed at > 48 hours. Based on this, a more appropriate research question to ask might be; 'what factors influence nurses' practices in the timing of changing IV tubing?' A question such as this has more clinical and theoretical relevance as it addresses the gap of why evidence-based recommendations are not being implemented rather than seeking to answer a question that already has been answered.

An alternative guide used by some researchers when formulating a research question is that of PICO. PICO stands for:

- Problem and/or Participants
- Intervention
- Comparison or Control
- Outcomes

PICO, however, is not necessarily applicable to all types of research studies. Rather, it has more relevance in guiding question formulation in certain types of studies, mainly those of randomised trials or prospective correlation studies (see Chapter 5 for further details). This is because some elements of PICO, such as the intervention and comparison or control components, have little relevance to studies which are descriptive or qualitative in nature. For studies that compare healthcare outcomes between two or more groups that are receiving different treatments, PICO is often recommended and used. For this reason, it is important for you to be familiar with its meaning as you may come across it when reading research papers. Table 3.2 exemplifies how using PICO can help define a research question.

Table 3.2   Use of PICO in formulating research questions

Problem, Participants	Intervention	Comparison	Outcomes	Research question
Preterm birth. Pregnant women at risk of preterm birth	Antibiotic therapy	No antibiotic therapy or placebo	Preterm birth	Does prophylactic antibiotic therapy, administered to women at risk of preterm birth, prevent preterm birth?

During the final stages of formulating a research question, a researcher must determine that the question is actually researchable. This is important to understand, as not all questions are amenable to study. For example, a question that asks 'should nurses work a thirteen hour clinical shift or an eight hour clinical shift?' is not a researchable question. This is because the question tends towards a value judgment, or simply put, it has the potential to elicit a 'yes/no' answer. Questions that tend towards 'yes/no' answers have limited relevance and provide minimal information for advancing healthcare theory or practice. Wood and Ross-Kerr (2006) suggest that a researchable research question must be an 'action' question. That is, a question that yields some hard facts that will explain, identify, evaluate, describe, explore or substantiate phenomena inherent to the problem under study.

Consider again the question 'should nurses work a thirteen hour clinical shift or an eight hour clinical shift?' You might brainstorm this topic and identify 'continuity of care' as an issue associated with clinical shift duration. The research problem might then be clarified as 'eight hour clinical shifts reduce continuity of care for healthcare clients compared to thirteen hour clinical shifts'. At this point, we don't know this for sure, rather, it is an issue of concern. The researchable research question might then be 'Do thirteen hour clinical shifts enable nurses to provide greater continuity of care than eight hour clinical shifts?' The action part of the question, that is the 'Do' stem, indicates that some type of investigation is warranted. This type of action question would require the researcher to explore the two types of clinical shifts and their impact on continuity of care. It would also lead the researcher to investigate whether one type of shift improves continuity of care over the other. It is because of these directional elements that we can now deem this type of question a researchable one.

Table 3.3 provides examples of researchable and non-researchable questions. Consider the difference between how these are phrased. Note down the action part of the researchable questions. Note how the non-researchable questions provide for yes/no answers whereas the researchable questions deem some form of investigation necessary.

Table 3.3   Example of non-researchable and researchable questions

Topic	Problem statement	Non-researchable question	Researchable question
Preterm birth	Preterm birth affects the psychological wellbeing of parents	Is preterm birth psychologically difficult for parents?	What is the psychological impact of preterm birth on parents who have a preterm baby?
Informed consent	Informed consent is essential in healthcare practice	Is informed consent a reality in clinical practice?	What are healthcare clients' understanding and experience of informed consent during healthcare provision?
Equal access to healthcare	Equal access to healthcare should be available to all	Is equal access to healthcare achievable?	What is the experience of differing groups in society in accessing their healthcare needs?

A further element in formulating a research question is to consider the type of question that must be asked to solve the research problem. Research questions can be described according to distinct types or levels depending on what the researcher wishes to find out. For example, research questions have been described as Level I, II and III, type questions (Wood & Ross-Kerr, 2006). Level I questions are questions that are formulated when there is little known about a topic of interest. The research question is posed to seek information or describe existing phenomena related to the subject area. In this sense, formulating a Level I question involves focusing on 'description' for solving the research problem. Level I questions are amenable to both quantitative and qualitative type of enquiries. An example of a Level I research questions might be: 'Does the use of the internet influence health service users' decision-making behaviours?' To answer this question a researcher would need to design a study that will describe attitudes, opinions, views or experiences. Level II

ACTIVITY 3.3

questions are formulated when there is some existing knowledge on a topic of interest but little understanding of the relationship between phenomena associated with the topic. Level II questions usually require quantitative type studies to effectively answer these because some type of statistical analysis is required to determine relationships. An example of a Level II type question is 'Do women who present with decreased fetal movements in the third trimester of pregnancy have increased adverse pregnancy outcomes?' To answer this question a researcher would need to design a study that will explore the relationship between decreased fetal movements and adverse pregnancy outcomes. Level III type questions are formulated when there is a considerable amount of information about the topic of interest. The question is formulated to test a theory or to examine whether there is a causal relationship between two or more variables. To effectively answer a Level III type question a quantitative study design, or more specifically, an experimental design, is required. An example of a Level III type question is 'Does cryotherapy relieve muscle soreness after exercise more effectively than muscle massage?' In this example, there may be knowledge that cryotherapy and massage (the variables) are beneficial for relieving post-exercise muscle soreness. The question is asked to determine whether one treatment relieves muscle soreness after exercise better than the other.

Once a research question has been clearly defined a final exercise before proceeding with the research study is to consider whether the question is feasible for study. What this means is that a researcher must ask him/herself whether it is possible to secure the necessary resources to conduct the study. It can often be the case that important research questions are formed that warrant exploration but the resources necessary to answer the question are not available. To determine if a research question is feasible a researcher will need to give some thought to the time required to answer the question, the costs that the study might incur, the available financial resources, the study location and the accessibility of the required study participants. Once the study has been confirmed as being feasible the next step for the researcher is to proceed with setting specific study aims and objectives.

Research Hypotheses

Before moving on to the research aim and objectives, it is important at this point to differentiate a research question from a research hypothesis. A research hypothesis, although closely related to a research question, goes somewhat further in that it suggests an answer to that question. It is written as a statement rather than a question in which the researcher offers a prediction as to what the outcome of the study will be. A research hypothesis (or prediction) is stated at the outset, the study is then conducted to test the hypothesis and the results of the study are said to either support the hypothesis or not to support it. Not all studies require a research hypothesis; rather they are usually developed for studies in which we wish to test some underlying theory.

Deciding on whether a research question or a research hypothesis will be used in a study is very much dependant on the type and purpose of the study. In some instances a researcher could observe possible associations between variables in clinical practice. For example, it might be observed that men who have epidural analgesia during prostate surgery appear to have fewer respiratory infections. A prediction, based on these observations, that men who have a general anaesthetic during prostate surgery have a higher incidence of respiratory infection, could then be made. This represents the initial stages of hypothesis development in that assumptions or some form of assumed knowledge is required. A formal research hypothesis, for testing in a study, is then further developed by the researcher, based on these assumptions.

In developing a research hypothesis, there are two types of hypotheses that must be considered.

The Null Hypothesis

The null hypothesis states that there is no difference between the particular groups or variables under investigation. Using the epidural example from above, the null hypothesis would state that 'there is no difference in the rate of respiratory infection in men who have epidural analgesia during prostate surgery and in men who have a general anaesthetic during prostate surgery'. The researcher would then need to design a study that tests this. If the results of the study show that there is no difference in respiratory infection rates irrespective of the method of analgesia, then the researcher concludes that the results of the study support the null hypothesis. Alternatively, if the results show that there is actually a difference, that is, the rate of respiratory infection is higher in men who have epidural analgesia compared to men who have a general anaesthetic (or vice-versa), then the researcher must conclude that the null hypothesis is not supported by the study results.

The Alternative Hypothesis

The alternative hypothesis states that there is a difference between the particular groups or variables under investigation with the direction of that difference provided. Using again the epidural example from above, in developing the alternative hypothesis a researcher would now state that 'the incidence of respiratory infection is lower in men who have epidural analgesia during prostate surgery than in men who have a general anaesthetic during prostate surgery'. The direction of the prediction is in favour of respiratory infection being lower in men who have epidural analgesia. As with the null hypothesis, the study is conducted to test this theory. If the results of the study demonstrate that men who have epidural analgesia have less respiratory infections than men who have a general anaesthetic then the researcher must conclude that the study results support the alternative hypothesis. If in fact men who have a general anaesthetic have a lower respiratory infection rate or if the study finds no difference in respiratory infection rates between the two groups, then the researcher must conclude that the alternative hypothesis is not supported by the study results. Table 3.4 provides some examples of research hypotheses.

Research Aim and Objectives

Once the research question or hypothesis has been clearly defined, the next step is to determine the research aim and to establish research objectives. The research aim

Table 3.4   Examples of research hypotheses

Research Problem	Null Hypothesis	Alternative Hypothesis
Progression-free survival in people with early stage Hodgkin lymphoma could be extended depending on the type of treatment administered	There is no difference in rates of progression-free survival in people with early stage Hodgkin lymphoma who receive chemotherapy plus radiotherapy compared to people who receive chemotherapy alone	Chemotherapy plus radiotherapy compared to chemotherapy alone, for early stage Hodgkin lymphoma, leads to increased rates of progression-free survival
Infection causes preterm birth	There is no difference in preterm birth rates in women who receive prophylactic antibiotic therapy compared to women who do not receive prophylactic antibiotic therapy	The incidence of preterm birth is lower in women who receive prophylactic antibiotic therapy than in women who do not receive prophylactic antibiotic therapy
Type of dressing affects the rate of healing of foot ulcers in people with diabetes	There is no difference in foot ulcer healing in people with diabetes when hydrogel wound dressings are used compared to alternative types of dressings.	Foot ulcers in people with diabetes heal more effectively when hydrogel dressings, compared to alternative dressings, are used

must arise directly from the research question (or hypothesis) and must be specific as it directs the remainder of the research study.

Many undergraduate healthcare students and novice researchers often find it difficult to differentiate between research aims and research objectives. This is not surprising considering that they are often used interchangeably in the literature and are synonymous in most dictionaries. In research studies, however, research aims and objectives are not one and the same, rather they represent two very distinct components that must be considered and described as such.

Research Aim

The research aim is a concise statement setting down the intent of a research study. It describes the overall purpose of the study and emphasizes the study's desired end accomplishment. Although some research studies might list a number of aims, it is recommended that a study should preferably have one or, at a maximum, two broad aims. The study's aim(s) may then be delineated further by identifying a number of associated objectives. When detailing a research aim it is recommended that researchers use strong verbs to do this as these provide a greater indication of the intent of the study. Examples of these include words such as evaluate, determine, explain and assess. Weak verbs, such as understand, consider and learn, for example, are not sufficient (or strong enough) when detailing the aim of a research study.

Research Objectives

Research objectives, on the other hand, are specific statements of purpose in which a research aim is broken down into more detailed and manageable sections (Moule &

Goodman, 2014). They should be consistent with the aim and must be realistic and achievable. Importantly they must not be a repetitive list of each other or an expression of the aim in different ways, rather, each objective should read as a single statement of intent as to how the various elements within the study's aim will be accomplished.

Determining appropriate research objectives can be a challenging task for many researchers (novice and experienced). This is because it is often difficult to separate out the elements of the overall aim. A useful aid to assist with this is the mnemonic SMART (Doran, 1981). SMART initially gained momentum in the business/corporate world (Meyer, 2003), however, it has now been adapted and applied to objective setting in a variety of settings including that of healthcare. SMART stands for:

1. Specific: be precise about what you are going to do
2. Measurable: you should know when you have reached your goal
3. Achievable: don't attempt too much
4. Realistic: do you have the necessary resources to achieve each objective?
5. Timely: be able to determine when each stage must be completed allowing for the possibility of potential delays.

As with the research aim, strong verbs are recommended when setting objectives. Table 3.5 provides examples of research aims and objectives. Note how each aim is concise and directly related to the research question. Note also how the objectives are numbered whereas the aim is written as a single sentence.

Table 3.5 Establishing research aims and objectives

Research Question	Aim	Objectives
What are current national practices for predicting and preventing preterm birth?	To determine current national maternity care practices for predicting and preventing preterm birth	1. To describe current national management strategies for predicting and preventing preterm birth 2. To determine similarities/differences in practices 3. To compare national practices with best practice recommendations 4. To compare national practices with the international literature and the empirical evidence base
What are burns victims' attitudes towards the psychological care they receive?	To determine current psychological care practices in people with burns from the perspective of these people	1. To determine the current types of psychological care received by people with burns 2. To identify potential deficits in psychological care provision from the perspectives of people with burns 3. To identify areas for improvement or development from the perspective of people with burns

Chapter Summary

The focus of this chapter was to provide some essential understandings of the initial stages that are required when undertaking a research study. From reading this chapter, you should have an understanding of the term research problem and the important place that it has when planning a research study. You should have a clear understanding of the term research question and of the need to clearly define this question prior to commencing a study. By reading this chapter, you should also have an understanding of research aims and objectives and be able to differentiate between them. Another important understanding that should have emerged for you from this chapter is an understanding of the time required in formulating a research question. It is very important for a researcher not to rush these crucial initial stages as this could have serious consequences for the study as it progresses. If a researcher does not spend some time developing and refining the research question, he/she may find, following study commencement, that the research question is not actually feasible for study, that it already has been answered or that it is too vague or underdeveloped to add anything of value to healthcare practice and/or theoretical advancement. Borrowing from the words of Leonardo da Vinci, a researcher who fails to define a clear research question and/or develop appropriate research aims and objectives is like '*a pilot who goes into a ship without rudder or compass and never has any certainty where he is going*' (Leonardo da Vinci, Notebooks, 1508–1515).

🔑 Key Points 🔑

- All research work begins by identifying a topic of interest for study.
- A research problem is something related to a topic of interest that is concerning, thought provoking or perplexing. It is something that must be solved. It is always declarative and not interrogative.
- A research question is one that is clearly defined, is researchable, is feasible and ultimately has relevance to clinical/theoretical healthcare practice.
- A research hypothesis is a statement in which a prediction on the outcome or results of a study is made.
- A research aim is a broad statement of the overall purpose of the study. It should emphasise the study's desired end accomplishment.
- Research objectives are specific statements of purpose in which a research aim is broken down into more detailed and manageable sections.

Useful Online Resources

www.who.int
http://handbook.cochrane.org
www.stats.gla.ac.uk/steps/glossary/hypothesis_testing

4

Searching and Reviewing the Literature

Introduction

Having identified a research problem or topic of interest, the next step is undertaking the literature review. A literature review may be defined as a critical synopsis of research studies and other works, which offer insights into the research problem and help to put it in context (Coughlan et al., 2013). It is important to recognise that a review is more than a simple summary, and that the literature should be critically appraised and presented in a manner that indicates that the reviewer recognises the strengths and limitations that exist within the studies.

Today, the term literature review encompasses a number of methods of gathering and presenting data from the literature. These literature reviews vary in their level of complexity from the traditional narrative reviews to in-depth systematic reviews. Similarly, the rationale for undertaking a literature review can also vary. A review, for example, may be undertaken to find a resolution to a clinical problem, or as part of research study, or it may be a research study in its own right as in the case of a systematic review. While literature reviews can vary in their complexity, there are similarities in how they are undertaken and the first step involves developing a search strategy so that literature that offers insights into the research problem / topic of interest can be identified.

☑ Learning Outcomes ☑

By the end of this chapter you should be able to:

- Describe the different types of literature review
- Recognise the different sources and types of literature
- Develop a search strategy
- Describe how to limit or expand a search.

Types of Literature Review

As mentioned earlier, there are different types of literature review which have different functions and so differing methodologies that determine how they are undertaken. Some of the different types of literature review have been included in the box below.

Examples of Types of Literature Review

- Narrative Review
- Systematic Review
- Integrative Review
- Scoping Review
- Concept Analysis.

Narrative Review

Before the advent of the systematic review, what is now described as the narrative or traditional review was the primary method of undertaking a literature review. While this type of review was and is expected to demonstrate a reasonably methodical review of the relevant literature, the argument is made that some narrative reviews are undertaken in an unsystematic manner without a review strategy being expressed (Aveyard, 2010) or they only present the literature supporting one side of an argument (Bettany-Saltikov, 2012). On the other hand, some narrative reviews were also undertaken in a systematic manner, with clear review strategies and searches that were systematic in nature. While the former type of narrative review is unacceptable from an academic perspective, the latter is a fundamental way of informing the science of many disciplines (Coughlan et al., 2013). However, despite the fact that the latter narrative reviews are undertaken in a methodical or systematic manner they should not be mistaken for systematic reviews which are methodologically different.

Narrative reviews are used in a number of ways. These include as literature reviews within theses or research proposals, they may be presented in their own right to offer an evidenced-based solution to a clinical problem, and they are often presented as an academic assignment. A good narrative review is expected to have a clearly identified research problem and search strategy, to critically appraise and synthesize the literature that is presented and to be replicable. While the search may not be as in-depth as in a systematic review, it should be methodical and should present alternative views on the topic being discussed. Depending on the purpose of a narrative review, the outcome may be a solution to, or clarification of the research problem and/or the development of a research question.

Systematic Review

A systematic review differs from a narrative review in that the focus of the literature search is on a specific research question (Bettany-Saltikov, 2012) rather than a research problem. It is regarded as being a research methodology in its own right (Clarke, 2006) and is expected to demonstrate a robust rigour throughout, to reduce the risk of biases occurring (Bettany-Saltikov, 2012). The difference between a narrative and systematic review can be seen in how the latter selects and manages studies. It is expected that the methodology used in a systematic review will be transparent and clearly describe how the reviewer plans to search for, select and evaluate the studies in the review. The aim should be to systematically seek out all studies, published and unpublished in order to present the most accurate overview of the research (Clarke, 2006) and reduce the risk of bias. It is not uncommon to find that the results of some studies are not published in the journals or other media. This can occur for any number of reasons including the results not being regarded as statistically significant, or because not all the findings had the expected outcome only part of the study was published. Nonetheless, the inclusion of these studies can help to ensure a more accurate summary of the research findings on this topic (Clarke, 2006). In selecting suitable studies to include within a review, the inclusion criteria will often identify the type of methodology (e.g. RCT - Randomised Control Trial) and sometimes the hypothesis that will make a study suitable for the review.

The results from a systematic review can be formulated in a number of different ways, depending on the type (design) of studies selected for the review. If the review selected studies that used experimental or quasi-experimental (see Chapter 5) designs then it may be possible to statistically integrate the findings of these studies using meta-analysis. If this is not possible then the evidence may be presented as a narrative synthesis, which involves presenting the findings in words. A meta-synthesis approach may be used to integrate findings from studies that gathered narrative (words) data (Polit & Beck, 2012).

While systematic reviews offer an approach that appears rigorous, it should be treated similarly to any other piece of research and critically appraised. The robustness of a systematic review is dependent on how well it was conducted and to what degree efforts were made to include all appropriate research. Bettany-Saltikov (2012) identifies limitations such as excluding works not published in English as one factor that can undermine the results of a systematic review.

Integrative Review

Systematic reviews often select studies with a specific methodology, and in a large number of cases the methodology selected is experimental in nature, namely in the form of randomised control trials. Integrative reviews were developed with the belief that reviews should be more inclusive and contain non-experimental methodologies, theoretical and conceptual literature as well as experimental research, in order to give a greater insight to the topic being reviewed (Whittemore & Knafl, 2005). Torraco (2005) states that integrative reviews fall into two types. The first type reviews the more mature topic that has a large volume of data and has been reviewed and discussed extensively. The role of the integrative review in this instance is to re-examine and critically analyse the literature that has developed around the topic and, in the light of this re-conceptualise, as appropriate, the ideas and beliefs that underpin the topic (Torraco, 2005). The second type relates to newer emergent topics. Torraco (2005) states that an integrative review of such a topic often leads to the development of a conceptual model or framework, particularly if the topic has not been subjected to a comprehensive review previously. Torraco (2005) adds that the expectation for both categories is that the reviewer will, through the conceptualisation or reconceptualization of the model or framework identify new perspectives on the topic.

While it may appear that an integrative review is similar to a narrative review, particularly if the latter is undertaken in a systematic manner, integrative reviews claim that it is the new perspectives that are identified through conceptualisation that differentiates it from the more descriptive narrative review (Torraco, 2005).

Scoping Review

A scoping review, also known as a scoping project and scoping study, as its name suggests, focuses on identifying the scope or range of literature that is available on a particular topic or broad research question. This literature can include both quantitative and qualitative research as well as policy and conceptual literature (Anderson et al., 2008). The resulting literature can, in some instances, be quite diverse and so reviewers undertake a mapping exercise to summarise the results. Scoping reviews can be regarded as falling into one of two broad groups: those that map the literature with or without the view of determining the expediency of undertaking a systematic review; and those in which a scoping review can be recognised as a review methodology in its own right (Arksey & O'Malley, 2005). Some of the reasons for undertaking a scoping review can be seen in the box below.

Some Reasons for Undertaking a Scoping Review

1. To map the quantity and variety of research that is available on a topic. The focus of a scoping review in this instance is to present a summary of the available research rather than describing the findings.
2. To establish if it is worthwhile doing a systematic review on a particular research question. In this case, the scoping review is undertaken to determine if there is sufficient research available on the topic and if this question has been reviewed previously and if there is value in proceeding further.
3. To produce a summary of the findings from the literature that could be disseminated among those who lack the time or resources to undertake this form of study.
4. To expose gaps in the literature through drawing conclusions from the existing literature.

(Arksey & O'Malley, 2005)

The steps in undertaking a scoping review were described by Arksey and O'Malley (2005) as:

- identifying a broad research question or area of interest
- identifying literature that is relevant to the review through a wide search of multiple literature sources

- selecting literature relevant to the research question
- charting data from the literature
- organising, mapping, summarising and reporting the results of the review
- consulting with consumers and practitioners (optional step).

Again, the initial steps in a scoping review are similar to other forms of literature review.

Concept Analysis

A concept is an image, which the mind uses to represent objects or phenomenon. For example, if you think of a tree, a mental image appears in your mind. However, it is non-specific in the sense that it could be an oak or a palm tree depending on contextual issues such as where you are from, or where you happen to be now. While there is a universal understanding of the concept of a tree, in healthcare there are numerous concepts whose meaning are less concrete and more contextual in nature. Among these are concepts such as self-care, compliance, reassurance, hope, and coping to name a few. Considering these concepts, the first thing that may be noticed is that their meaning may differ depending on if you are a healthcare professional or a consumer of healthcare. It is therefore important to recognise that there are potentially different meanings to concepts depending on the context in which they are experienced.

A concept analysis may be defined as a process by which a concept that is of interest to a profession is studied to determine its attributes and characteristics (Cronin et al., 2010) in order to achieve a better understanding of that concept. There are a number of approaches to undertaking a concept analysis including Walker and Avant's (2011) method and Rodgers' Evolutionary Method (Rodgers & Knafl, 2000). Once the concept for analysis has been identified, the next step is to identify and collect literature related to that concept.

While the different types of literature review vary in their methodologies and outcomes, they all share a common function in that they need to search and identify literature that is appropriate to their review. While this chapter will focus mainly on searching from a narrative review perspective, aspects that pertain to other types of review will also be included.

Identifying Literature Sources

Literature can be obtained from a number of different sources. The most common source of literature utilised in reviews is published material in the form of books or journal articles. However, other sources of information exist such as unpublished literature, and reports from alternative media sources, for example television or radio, which can also be used. When undertaking a review of the literature the reviewer should ideally aim to use as many search methods and literature sources as possible to ensure that the search is systematic in nature. Greenhalgh and Peacock (2005) claim that there is a risk of missing important studies due to circumstances such as poor literature indexing, and multiple search methods and sources reduce this risk. There are a number of literature sources and some of these are included in the box below.

Sources of Literature

- Electronic databases
- Internet search engines
- Catalogues
- Grey literature

  - Conference proceedings
  - Unpublished literature (including PhD or Master thesis)

- Textbooks and dictionaries
- Manual searches.

Database and Internet Searches

The most common method of undertaking a literature search is online, using databases and search engines which are major sources of literature and information for both reviewers and researchers. Databases are compilations of literature in an electronic format. The literature is derived from a variety of sources such as journals, books, dissertations and conferences to name a few, and depending on level of access the reader can retrieve abstracts, references or full texts of the articles selected in the search. While some databases will offer free access, a membership subscription is usually required for full text access. Establishments such as universities, third level colleges and organisations such as hospitals normally have institutional subscriptions to one or more databases which can be accessed by staff and students linked to that institution. A selection of useful databases can be found in Table 4.1.

Table 4.1   A selection of electronic databases

Database	Main Content	Type of Access
Allied and Complementary Medicine Database (AMED)	Literature related to allied health literature, complementary medicine and palliative care	Subscription required
British Nursing Index (BNI)	Nursing literature, mainly of UK origin	Subscription required
Centre for Reviews and Dissemination (CRD)	Systematic reviews and meta-analysis for evidence-based medicine	Free access
Cochrane Library	Database of systematic reviews	Free access
Cumulative Index to Nursing and Allied Health Literature (CINAHL)	Literature related to nursing and allied health issues.	Subscription required

(Continued)

Table 4.1   (Continued)

Database	Main Content	Type of Access
Joanna Briggs Institute	Evidence-based research related to nursing and allied healthcare	Subscription required
Proquest Nursing and Allied Health Source	Covers literature related to nursing, allied health, complementary and alternative medicine including physical and occupational therapy, and rehabilitation.	Subscription required
PsycINFO	This database contains peer-reviewed literature related to mental health and the behavioural sciences	Subscription required
PubMed/MEDLINE	A database of literature related to life sciences, particularly biomedicine. Free access to this database is available through PubMed	Free access
Social Care Online	This site offers access to UK government documents and reports, and journal articles related to social care and social work	Free access

(Adapted from Coughlan et al., 2013)

Literature stored on databases can be accessed by topic or author. The latter is useful if you know a particular author writes a great deal on a specific topic. The former is the more customary way of searching using a database. Topics are accessed through the use of keywords, which are words, terms or phrases that are used by database providers to index the works that they have stored. Keywords are discussed in more detail later in the chapter.

Search engines are computer programs that can enable a user to search for specific information on the internet. The result of the search is presented as a 'webpage' which offers links to a series of sites that are deemed to match the search parameters. There are numerous search engines (AoL, Ask, Bing, Dogpile, Google, Google Scholar) and results from the different engines can vary, as each uses its own unique software programme to trawl through the web. Therefore, it can be worthwhile utilising a number of different search engines.

Search engines are often used to search for published documents and reports from state and international agencies, and voluntary and professional bodies. They can also offer access to databases and alternative websites. However, when surfing the web for information, it is worth remembering that webpages can contain unsupported and sometimes inaccurate commentaries, so it is important to critically read the information presented and where possible, to use recognised, trustworthy sites only (Ely & Scott, 2007).

Catalogues

With the advent of electronic databases, catalogue searches have almost been relegated to a thing of the past. Catalogues were hard copy indices that stored the publications of a profession by author and topic. CINAHL, for example, was originally a catalogue index before becoming an electronic database. Catalogues only reflected the annual published content so a search involved reviewing each year of the catalogue in order to identify literature. By today's standards such a search would be regarded as cumbersome and time-consuming. However, there are instances where such a search may need to be undertaken. Researchers who undertake historical research or are looking for older studies may need to undertake catalogue searches. Rebar et al. (2011) state that most of the electronic databases only hold literature published after 1982, and while MEDLINE does contain literature back to the 1940s, generally any searches that predate 1982 will involve a manual search of this medium.

Grey Literature

While the vast majority of literature is available through the different electronic databases, there is some literature that is more obscure and therefore less accessible. This literature is known as Grey Literature and includes unpublished Masters dissertations and PhD theses, conference reports, publications in obscure journals, or some e-journals and unpublished reports (Grove et al., 2013). At undergraduate and master's degree level there is a tendency to simply stick to the published, peer-reviewed articles that are available in the more commonly used electronic databases. However, this approach can lead to a 'publication bias', especially in the case of systematic reviews, if non-published studies and literature are excluded (Polit & Beck, 2012). This is because studies with significant findings are more likely to be published in leading journals, and those with less significant or negative findings are more likely to be rejected (Grove et al., 2013). Thus, relying on only the main literature sources can lead to a situation where alternative views and findings can be overlooked.

The main reason for not including grey literature is that it can be difficult to access. Universities and third-level institutions usually have databases that will identify dissertations and theses generated in their own establishments. These are usually available to students of that institution on request, and sometimes by interlibrary loan to readers in another third level institution. Other information on the grey literature is available at GreyNet (www.greynet.org) and the Index to Theses database (www.theses.com).

Textbooks and Dictionaries

Another useful source of information is books. The majority of books are available as hard copy texts but newer editions and new books are usually available as e-books that can be purchased for download. Books can offer a background on the topic that has been selected and are often the initial reading on the subject. However, books need to be read with the understanding that the research evidence they contain can be dated even at publication, as 12 months or more can have elapsed between the book being written and published.

When searching for books, university or college library catalogues are often a good place to start and these will usually indicate if an electronic copy of the book is available to readers. Libraries are also good sources of older books which can offer a historical perspective on the topic being studied. Dictionaries and thesauruses can be helpful for defining terms and concepts, and can prove useful when attempting to identify keywords.

Manual Searches

Manual exploration of the literature is usually undertaken to complement database and other searches, and to ensure that no significant material has been missed or omitted. There are a number of methods used to manually search for literature and those included here are by no means exclusive.

One of the simplest methods is called an ancestry search (Grove et al., 2013) and involves checking the reference lists of the articles that have been obtained to identify literature not already reviewed. This is a particularly useful method where the articles already acquired are recently published and have reasonably up-to-date reference lists. Another method is known as a descendent search. Some databases and search engines such as Web of Science and Google Scholar will allow a reader to track seminal articles on the topic of interest to see who has cited them as these works are also likely to be of interest.

Literature reviews on the topic of interest can be another way of identifying studies in more obscure journals. However, it is important, whenever possible, to secure the original work, rather than depending on a secondary author to accurately describe or critically review the work. The only way to ensure an accurate commentary on a study is to review the original article or what is called the primary source. A reviewer should only cite from an author who makes reference to a primary source (a secondary source), if the primary work is inaccessible.

As mentioned earlier, an author search may be undertaken if there is an author who writes extensively on the topic of interest. It can sometimes be difficult to identify such authors until a topic search is undertaken.

Sifting through research journals can be another way of identifying articles of interest. This can especially be the case if the topic is in a specialist area that is supported by dedicated journals such as Cancer Care or Mental Health. This type of search is often tedious and time consuming as it can involve selecting the content index from each issue and checking to see if there are articles that relate to the topic of interest.

Searching and Retrieving the Literature

An important feature of research is that it should to a large degree be replicable. In order to achieve this, at the level of a literature review, it is essential that the reader can follow the steps of the search. It is therefore important to make good notes in preparation for writing up the search methodology. While the methodology may never produce exactly the same result, it should be at least able to locate the same literature. Information that the reader will require includes the databases and keywords used and other search methods used. An example of how a literature search might be documented can be seen in a review by McMahon and Fleury (2012) who described their search in relation to falls risks (see box, p. 47).

Documenting the Literature Search

Systematic computer searches were conducted in 2010 using PsycINFO, PubMed, CINAHL, and the Cochrane Review databases (2000–2010). Search terms included: falls; accidental falls, fall prevention, nursing, physical activity intervention, exercise intervention, physical activity. Reference lists from relevant studies and resources were also reviewed to identify studies not found via computer search.

Source: McMahon and Fleury (2012: 2142)

While the advent of electronic databases has made literature searching seem a lot more straightforward, it is important to remember that the search should be performed in a systematic manner and is not just a case of identifying a few articles. Undertaking a systematic search is a skill that has to be learned and honed and is not something that always comes easy to novice researchers. Identifying the main beliefs and theories that support the research problem or question and being able to categorise these into keywords can make the process a lot easier (Lahlafi, 2007). Help from experts in the area and from specialist librarians can be useful in achieving this. They may also be able to recommend which databases and literary sources might be most beneficial to the search.

The principles of searching the different databases are reasonably similar, although there are some minor variations. Journal collections do vary between professional databases so it is better not to be limited to just one database. EBSCOhost offers access to a number of databases including CINAHL. On accessing a database such as CINAHL through EBSCOhost the searcher is offered a screen with a number of choices which can be found directly beneath the 'search' box, similar to the example in Figure 4.1.

The default screen opens to a basic search with 'search options' activated and in some instances a tick box 'suggest subject terms' may appear above the search box. The basic search is the simplest method of searching and involves inserting a keyword or phrase into the search box and selecting search. Search options offer the opportunity to limit or expand the search as necessary. If the 'suggest subject terms' box is ticked it will further define the search term, which can be useful if the term being used is broad and needs refining. Both these options can be switched off by simply clicking on 'Search Options' and the box for subject terms.

The simple search is ideal for single keywords. However, phrases can be regarded by the simple search as individual keywords and so the database is searched for all articles that include any of the words in the phrase. This can lead to a large number of hits, many which may not be related to the topic of interest. One way of managing this is to use parentheses ( ) or double commas " " to enclose the search term and thus identify to the database that these words should be considered as single keyword, for example (HIV and AIDs), see Figure 4.2. Another solution is the advanced search mode which offers an approach in which up to 12 search terms can be used together to either clarify, limit or expand the search. Combining keywords is accomplished through the use of what are called Boolean Operators, and this combining of keywords can also limit or expand the scope of the search. Boolean Operators will be discussed in more detail later in the chapter. When using advanced searches, the field of the search can also be

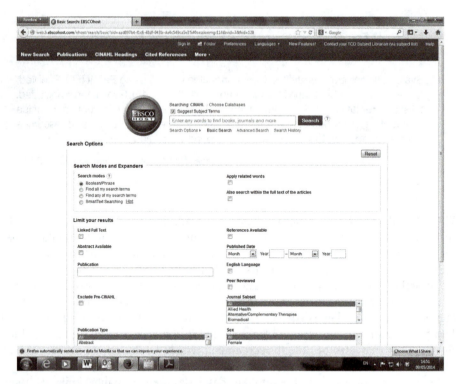

Figure 4.1   EBSCOhost search page

refined to allow for a number of different search options, such as single or multiple author searches, or to search for keywords within particular journals or in particular parts of an article, for example in the abstract. This can be accessed by opening the 'select a field' drop down box which is beside each keyword entry.

When undertaking a topic search it is important to identify the most applicable keywords to ensure that the most relevant works are accessed. The topic being searched may be indexed under a number of different headings, and while some articles may appear under all headings, others may not. Also, EBSCOhost allows searchers to search multiple databases simultaneously, and different databases may index articles using different headings. Consequently, to ensure the search is systematic, it is important to use different keywords. Most databases have a thesaurus or glossary of indexing terms that an individual undertaking a search can access, and this can help to identify the most common terms used. One of the more common indices for medical terms is MeSH (Medical Subject Headings) which is used by MEDLINE/PubMed. Another way of identifying alternative or unconventional keywords can be through discussing the topic with subject and clinical experts. It is also worthwhile reviewing the keywords that authors apply to their articles; these are often identified after the abstract.

Another issue that should be considered is spelling and terminology. Both MEDLINE and CINAHL are United States (US) databases and so use US spelling, which in some instances can vary from the English; words such as anaemia (anemia), haemophilia (hemophilia) and oesophagus (esophagus) are common examples. While databases do use word recognition software in an attempt to overcome this, it is still a good idea to search using the alternative spelling especially if using multiple databases. Terminology can also vary between different countries, for example, 'Emergency Room', 'Casualty'

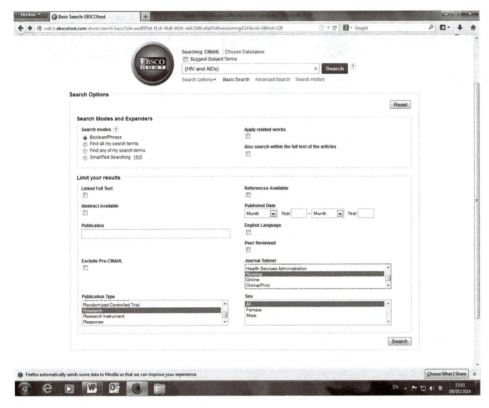

Figure 4.2   Search using parentheses

and 'Accident and Emergency' and again to ensure a systematic search it is shrewd to use the different terms as keywords.

After completing the initial searches the next step is to combine the searches. This allows the searcher to group all the results together rather than having to look at all the different searches. It also has the benefits of removing duplicate articles that are identified in the different searches. To do this the searcher selects 'search history', which will identify the results of the different searches. The searcher can then decide which searches will be combined.

Boolean, Truncation and Wildcard Operators

Boolean Operators

Both advanced searches and combining of basic searches are undertaken using Boolean operators. These commands are used to combine or exclude articles that contain particular keywords. The most commonly used Boolean operators are OR, AND and NOT and are written using block capitals. An example of how the number of hits can be expanded or limited using Boolean operators can be seen in Figure 4.3.

The initial search used the keyword HIV and AIDs, and had a very large number of hits (18,246) which needed to be refined. The Boolean AND was used to restrict the search. This ensured that both keywords were included in any article identified

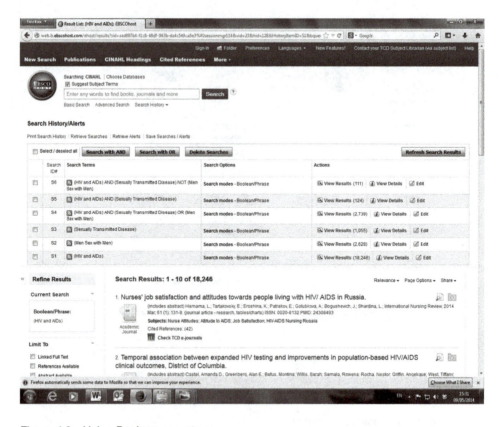

Figure 4.3   Using Boolean operators

> (HIV and AIDs) AND (Sexually Transmitted Disease) [STD]

and if only one of the terms was present then the article was excluded. The Boolean OR was then used to see the effect that including another keyword would have. In this instance the articles in the initial search result that included the keyword STD or MSM were included. This approach increased the number of hits by a large amount.

> (HIV and AIDs) AND (Sexually Transmitted Disease) OR (Men Sex with Men) [MSM]

It was then decided to exclude MSM altogether, so the Boolean NOT was used.

> (HIV and AIDs) AND (Sexually Transmitted Disease) NOT (Men Sex with Men)

The outcome was that articles containing the keywords "HIV and AIDs" and "Sexually Transmitted Disease" were identified but not if they included the keyword "Men Sex with Men". This final search identified 111 articles.

Truncation and Wildcard Operators

Truncation operators use the derivation of a keyword to identify and include other forms of the keyword in a search. The trunk of the keyword is followed directly by an asterisk which tells the database to use all keywords starting with this stem. An example using the term diet* will initiate a search for terms such as dietary and dietetic. However, it will also include dietician in the search terms which may not be a desired keyword.

Wildcards are search aids whereby a symbol is used to replace a letter. When a question mark is used to replace a letter the database will replace the symbol with all appropriate letters, for example wom?n will initiate a search for woman and women. Another wildcard is the hash symbol. This is used where an alternative spelling exists. The hash is used as the letter that may or may not be included in the spelling, for example a search for the term an#emia will search for both anaemia and anemia.

Boolean operators are standard on most databases but truncation and wildcards can vary between databases. It is always worthwhile therefore when undertaking a search to seek advice and discuss search strategies with the local librarian who will be in a position to offer guidance on the databases available.

Limiting the Search

Despite using a focused search, quite frequently the number of publications identified in a search can be relatively large. Managing this can be very challenging especially if there is a limited time frame in which the work must be completed or a limited word

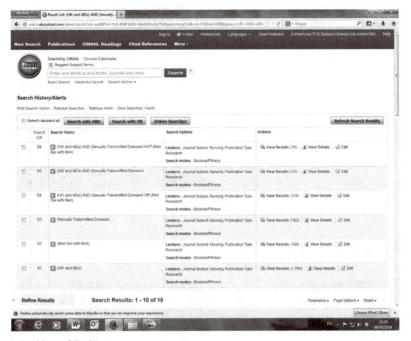

Figure 4.4   Use of limiters

count. In order to reduce the number of publications to be reviewed to more manageable numbers it may be necessary to limit the search parameters. As mentioned earlier, Boolean operators can be used to limit the terms within the search but it may still be necessary to impose further limits. A number of study limiters are available and in an EBSCOhost search they appear when 'search options' is highlighted. The effect of using the limiters 'Publication Type: Research' and 'Journal Subset: Nursing' (see Figure 4.2) can be seen when comparing the results from Figure 4.3 with Figure 4.4.

Publications can be limited by the age of the study. This involves setting date parameters. Conventions for academic assignments usually expect publications to be recent origin, within the last five to ten years. There are exceptions to this, such as historical research or where a study is regarded as being seminal to the research area. In some instances, the topic being studied may have a dearth of recent literature, and it may be necessary to include a larger number of older publications. In situations such as this the reason for including older studies should be identified.

Publications can also be limited to peer-reviewed, research studies. Peer review and research are two separate limiters so one or both can be applied. In a literature review it is expected that the majority of publications included are research based. However, other publications are useful for adding context so it may be important to consider this when limiting the search. Depending on the database being used, studies in a number of different languages may be included in the search findings. Limiting publications to the English language can be another useful way of reducing the number of publications to be reviewed.

When limiting a search it is important to consider that there may be consequences. Limiting a search to full text articles, for example, may be useful if the reviewer only has access to the articles offered by the databases being searched. However, as third level institutions and colleges usually have subscriptions to numerous online journals limiting a search in this manner may remove the opportunity to review these publications. Another disadvantage can be that significant studies can fall outside the search parameters.

Evaluating the Search Strategy

When undertaking a literature review it is important to regularly reassess the research strategy. It is important to remember multiple searches are usually necessary when systematically reviewing the literature, so reviewing the effectiveness of the keywords and databases being used is important. Depending on the amount of literature being identified it may be necessary to broaden or narrow the search parameters. It is also important to regularly consider if the search terms correspond with the topic being reviewed. Otherwise there is a risk that the search may deviate into an unrelated theme.

Organising the Literature

Once the literature search has been undertaken the next step involves identifying which studies are pertinent to the review. The suitability of studies will depend on the type of review being undertaken and the focus of the review. Depending on the amount of literature identified in the search, it may not be possible to do an in-depth evaluation of each article. It can be useful at this stage to quickly scan sections of an article such as the abstract, introduction and discussion to see if it meets the criteria for inclusion. Sometimes it may be possible to identify whether an article is relevant from reading the abstract alone, especially as the reviewer becomes more familiar with the topic.

After determining which works will be included in the review, the next steps involve analysing and synthesising the literature. Grove et al. (2013) state that analysis can be subdivided into critical appraisal of the individual studies and then an evaluation of how the included studies differed or were similar in regard to how the studies were conducted, and results they found. There are numerous instruments available for critically appraising the robustness of research studies, either online (Critical Appraisal Skills Programme [CASP], 2010), in journals (Coughlan et al., 2007) or in textbooks (Polit & Beck, 2012). However, it must be remembered that a critical analysis is more than a collection of critiques and this is where comparing and contrasting of studies facilitates the outcome. It can be used to demonstrate how different methodological approaches offer distinctive perspectives on the topic, compare and contrast results between studies, highlight the strengths and limitations of the different approaches and identify any gaps in the literature. It is through the analysis of the literature that a reviewer begins to comprehend and connect the different theories and concepts in the literature and begins to clarify these and formulate a research question or outcome to the review. This clarification and formulation of ideas is known as synthesis.

Writing the Literature Review

The key element when writing a review, or any academic paper, is to present it in a logical manner so that the reader can understand how the work has been structured. The review should be presented in a clear and consistent style that demonstrates the writer's knowledge of the topic. The usual format consists of an introduction to the review, the presentation of the literature and finally a summary / conclusion. The format will vary to some degree depending on the purpose and type of review being undertaken. Usually the review consists of between one quarter and one third of the available word count in a research study (Brett Davis, 2007).

Introduction

In the introduction the reviewer identifies the purpose of the review and may offer some background in relation to the research problem. A description of the literature search should also be presented including the keywords and databases used, other search strategies employed, and any limitations to the search. Information on how the literature will be presented can also be useful here (Grove et al., 2013).

Presenting the Literature

It is in this section that the results of the search are presented and analysed. Remember this section should not simply be a description of the original authors' work, nor should it be a series of studies being critically analysed. The reviewer needs to present the literature in such a manner that the reader can identify what has been discovered and which findings appear to be from studies with rigorous methodologies and which studies appear to have limitations. If subheadings or themes are used to present the literature these should not stand in isolation. There should be continuity between the different sections so that the reader understands how each section links with the previous section.

It is important to remain objective and impartial when presenting the findings of or analysing studies. It is important therefore to support observations on the strengths or limitations of a study, with reference to research textbooks or articles. It is also important to present both sides of an argument. For example, studies that do not support the planned hypothesis as well as those that do, should be presented in the review (Polit & Beck, 2012).

Summary / Conclusion

This section draws the literature review to a close. It usually commences by summarising what has been discovered in relation to the topic being studied and any gaps in the literature that have been identified. The reviewer usually concludes with recommendations that are drawn from what has been found. These can include how the review may be used to improve practice, or how it supports the need for the research in the proposed study to be undertaken.

Referencing

If the literature review is a stand-alone piece of work then the reference list will be included here. However, if the review is part of a bigger study, then the reference list will be left until the end of the work. All the studies mentioned in the review should have their full bibliographical reference included in the reference list. This allows the reader to source the original work.

Chapter Summary

There are different types of literature reviews, with varying levels of complexity, ranging from the classical narrative review to the systematic review. However, all forms share common features in that there is a need to search for and gather literature related to their chosen topic. While the depth and methodology underpinning the review may vary, the principles of performing a search remain similar.

Searching for literature can be time consuming and in some instances frustrating, particularly where there appears to be too little or an overwhelming amount of available literature. Refining, limiting and expanding searches are important skills in overcoming these difficulties, as well as recognising why these difficulties arise.

A literature review can be described as a discourse between the reviewer and the reader. It is therefore important that the reader is assisted to understand the significance of the results from the literature as well as the implications for practice and patient care. Consequently, it is important that the reviewer can offer a critical analysis of the studies presented as well as being able to assimilate the results to offer an understanding to the reader. Finally, these results need to be written and presented to the reader, in a manner that is clear and logical.

🔑 Key Points 🔑

- There are a number of different types of literature review including: narrative, systematic, integrative and scoping reviews, and concept analysis.
- A literature review can be a stand-alone piece of work or may be a part of a research study.
- Narrative reviews undertaken in a systematic manner are not systematic reviews.
- There are many sources from which literature can be gathered including: databases and catalogues, grey literature and text books.
- Keywords are used to access the database index so that the relevant literature can be identified.
- The most common Boolean operators are OR, AND, and NOT.
- Critical analysis and synthesis of the literature are essential parts of a literature review.

5

Getting to Grips with Research Designs

Introduction

This chapter presents an overview of a number of research designs that are used in healthcare research. We have classified these designs as experimental, quasi-experimental and non-experimental (see Table 5.1). The non-experimental designs are further divided into those that collect numerical data and those that focus on words or narrative data (see Table 5.2).

The characteristics of each research design are outlined and their relevance to the practical endeavour of undertaking a study is explained. This will help you decide when reading papers if the research questions posed fit with the chosen design. It is important to note that the exploration of methodologies and designs in this chapter is not exhaustive and the reader may want to explore more specialist texts for additional detail.

☑ Learning Outcomes ☑

By the end of this chapter you should be able to:

- Outline the main characteristics of the principal research designs used in healthcare research
- Describe the characteristics of experimental, quasi-experimental and non-experimental (numbers and words) studies
- Identify the features of paradigms that underpin the various research designs
- Explain how the characteristics of a chosen research design impacts on the research process.

Table 5.1   Classification of research designs

Experimental Designs	True Experiment
	Quasi-experiment
Non-experimental designs (Numerical)	Descriptive
	Correlational
	Causal-comparative/ex-post facto
Non-experimental designs (Narrative/ Words)	Descriptive
	Phenomenology
	Ethnography
	Grounded Theory
	Narrative
	Action Research
	Case Study*

*Case study is presented in the second part of this chapter but it is recognised that such a study may equally be undertaken using numerical and/or narrative data.

Paradigms

As outlined in Chapter 3, the starting point for any research is identifying a topic of interest following which a problem statement, research question or hypothesis, aim(s) and objectives are developed. The next step is to choose a research design that is best suited to answering the question posed. All research designs have certain characteristics that define them and distinguish them from each other and researchers must have some understanding of these in order to make sure they choose the design that is congruent with the purpose of their study.

Most researchers come with an idea of what they want to find out and to a certain degree the type of data they want to collect. They will also have ideas about what constitutes knowledge and the type of research that is undertaken to develop it. These ideas are often reflective of their shared beliefs with the community of scientists of which they are members. These beliefs or modes of thinking have been categorised into a number of paradigms (see Chapter 1), which direct the type of research that is undertaken. This means that in aligning themselves with a particular paradigm, researchers will tend to adopt study designs that are congruent with it.

Commonly cited paradigms include positivism, post-positivism, interpretivism/ constructivism, critical/transformative/participatory/advocacy and others such as naturalist, realist, emancipatory and post-modernist. The beliefs inherent in the most prominent of these in healthcare research are presented so that you can achieve some insight into how they influence researchers' approaches to the conduct of their studies. These will include positivism, post-positivism, interpretivism/constructivism and critical/transformative/participatory/advocacy.

That is not to say that you may not encounter the 'others' in your reading or research that 'cut across' paradigms. However, it is impossible in a text of this nature to address the ever-shifting nature of paradigms that are apparent in contemporary research and knowledge development. We recognise also that the interchangeable use of terms in the literature to describe the range of paradigms can be confusing. Nonetheless, what is important is that researchers should clearly outline the paradigm that underpins their study or why they might have a foot in more than one camp. By doing so, the reader can judge if the conduct of the study 'fits' within the realms of the chosen paradigm thereby facilitating analysis of its overall quality.

Positivism/Post-positivism

Positivism, in various guises has been a dominant mode of thinking for many centuries but for our purposes its fundamental influence in research is that it underpins the traditional or scientific method referred to in Chapter 1. Positivist principles included belief in the existence of an objective reality and that it is possible for the researcher to be objective. Also, observation and measurement are fundamental, establishing cause and effect (*a* causes *b*) is feasible and generalising results and establishing laws is achievable. Positivists attempted to mirror the methods used in the natural sciences, for example physics and chemistry. Ultimately, however, positivism was criticised and rejected because laws about human behaviour cannot be generated in the same way as they can for objects in the natural world. As a result, what is known as post-positivism emerged as a new philosophical tradition.

Post-positivism has retained aspects of positivism but it is considered more moderate. For instance, prediction, generalisation, measurement, observables and researcher objectivity continue to be hallmarks of post-positivist philosophy. However, there are differences in how these features are interpreted. For example, there is acknowledgement that while some predictions about humans and their behaviour can be made it is impossible to predict that they will behave in a certain way in every situation. Human beings are individuals who are unique, unpredictable and often not representative of the group to which they belong. Therefore, researchers in the post-positivist tradition, develop strategies for managing and controlling these differences (Routledge, 2007). Similarly, generalisations are valued but it is recognised that these are dependent on the context in which they happen. Aspects of human behaviour that are observable and can be measured continue to be important but it is now conceded that phenomena that are *unobservable* (feelings, behaviours) exist also. Researcher objectivity in the process of conducting research continues to be a key factor but it is accepted that none of us is truly objective. We are inherently biased by our values and beliefs, cultural experiences and way of looking at the world. With this awareness, researchers in the post-positivist tradition develop strategies such as repeated testing to ensure their interpretations are as objective as possible. Thus, knowledge and theories that are developed are approximately true and absolute truth cannot be achieved.

In healthcare research, experimental, quasi-experimental and non-experimental studies that collect numerical data adhere in varying degrees to the tenets of positivism and post-positivism. Characteristics that are likely to be features of these studies are outlined in the box below.

Features of Research Studies Underpinned by Positivism/Post-positivism

- Systematic inquiry – the scientific method
- Scientists are influenced by their interests, cultural experiences, world views
- Observation and measurement – phenomena are reduced to entities that can be measured
- Multiple measures and observations (repeated testing/replication)
- Control (of variables that may interfere)
- Knowledge generation through explanation and description
- Objective knowledge can be gained from direct observation and experience but it is fallible and subject to revision by repeated measures
- Large sample sizes
- Generalise results to the wider population in a given context
- Determining the probability that a hypothesis is true/false (not proving)
- Development of theories that can only be approximately (probably) true.

Interpretivism/Constructivism

Although there are those who would suggest that interpretivism and constructivism are distinct from each other (Andrews, 2012; Ross, 2012) they are often described together. Interpretivism/constructivism emerged as a critique of positivism. The central belief is that human beings' reality is constructed through the meanings they develop as a result of their experiences and their interactions with others in a social world. Simply stated, a person's values and beliefs about the world are influenced by their experiences of that world and the people with whom they interact. There is recognition that in any given situation, multiple perspectives exist. For example, this acknowledges that the perspective of a healthcare professional may and is likely to be different to that of a patient or client availing of a service.

Interpretivist/constructivist research seeks to understand the world of human experience from the perspective of the person experiencing it. The aim is to uncover the meanings they attach to those experiences. These meanings are revealed most often through engagement and interaction with the participants in a study. The context in which people construct their reality is fundamental and the interpretivist/ constructivist researcher often explores the daily living and experiences of the participants in order to better understand. The purpose is not to seek cause and effect relationships but to interpret the meanings the participants have of the world.

The role of researchers is often described as collaborative and they are integral to the research process. They do not stand 'outside' the research but are involved throughout. They are acknowledged also as subjective beings who have constructed their reality and attached meaning through their personal, social and cultural experiences. Researchers recognise how their own reality impacts on how they interpret the world of the participants in the study. The outcome of researchers' interpretations is patterns or themes and possibly theories that are context specific and which cannot be generalised to other people or settings.

The interpretivist/constructivist paradigm has not 'replaced' positivism/post-positivism. Rather, they are complementary in that they generate different types of knowledge that ultimately contribute to our overall evidence base. However, that research in the interpretivist/constructivist tradition is still less highly regarded is apparent in the evidence-based practice movement. Healthcare research that is congruent with positivism/post-positivism such as the randomised controlled trial remains the gold standard and highest form of evidence while qualitative research or that which is aligned with interpretivism/constructivism is classed as much lower in the hierarchy. While there has been some recognition lately that results of interpretivist/constructivist-based research is gaining ground it is still regarded as supplementary to positivist/post-positivist-based research.

In healthcare research, non-experimental studies that collect narrative data (words) often adhere to the beliefs of interpretivism/constructivism. These can include but are not exclusive to qualitative descriptive/exploratory, phenomenology and narrative, and in some ethnographic, grounded theory and case study research. Characteristics that are likely to be features of these studies are outlined in the box below.

Features of Research Studies Underpinned by Interpretivism/Constructivism

- Aim to understand the perspective of the individuals in the study – focussed on the person who is experiencing
- Knowledge is developed through description, exploration, understanding and interpretation
- Small samples
- Context and situation specific
- Active involvement of participants as 'co-researchers'
- Researcher involved in the participants' world
- Interactive data collection methods
- Interpret words to gain understanding
- Outcomes are patterns of meaning, themes or theory
- Generalisable results are not an aim.

Critical/Transformative/Participatory/Advocacy

The third paradigm considered here is considered a critique of others for their failure to focus on questioning or transforming the existing situation. The labelling of this paradigm in this text as critical/transformative/participatory/advocacy is intentional in order to highlight how similar ideas have been characterised in the literature. However, we do acknowledge that each may have distinguishing features. Critical theorists have been concerned with social conditions and a critique of the known structure of society. They argue that reality is constructed through language and over time so that the existing social structures such as the way society, politics, culture, economy, gender and ethnicity are organised come to be seen as normal. They suggest that groups within society who are in power have a political agenda such as maintaining the status quo, which compromises the interests of other groups in society. Critical theorists believe in making people aware of what is happening so that the prevailing ideology can be challenged and other voices can be heard. According to Creswell (2009), those who subscribe to the advocacy and participatory world view have drawn on the work of the critical theorists in developing their focus on the concepts of enablement, empowerment and emancipation.

The critical/transformative/participatory/advocacy paradigm shares some features with interpretivism/constructivism. However, at the heart of this paradigm are social justice issues such as oppression, empowerment and inequality, and marginalised and/or oppressed groups often form the focus of research. In addition, there may be a political agenda and an action programme for reform may be evident. Consequently, the setting or context in which the research is taking place is fundamental. Collaboration is central and the researcher works *with* the participants so that they are not marginalised further. The research is seen as potentially empowering as it gives a voice to disenfranchised groups. For example, feminist and disability theory have been particularly associated with this paradigm.

In healthcare research, participatory action research is seen as being congruent with the critical/transformative/participatory/advocacy paradigm as it has a built-in commitment to action. Characteristics that are likely to be features of these studies are outlined in the box below.

Features of Research Studies Underpinned by Critical/ Transformative/Participatory/Advocacy Paradigm

- Aim to change a situation by challenging the current situation and planning change (action agenda for reform)
- Questions/issues are concerned with important social issues of the day e.g. oppression, empowerment, inequality, etc.
- Research inquiry needs to be intertwined with politics and a political agenda
- Working with others
- Collaborating through all stages of the research
- The researcher is embedded in the research group
- Highly contextualised knowledge.

Experimental Designs

Experimental designs, as the name suggests, involve 'experiments'. We may think of experiments as something that happens in a laboratory but experimentation is a common feature of all of our lives whether we are consciously aware of it or not. For example, if we decide that we want to get fitter we might try cycling as a means of doing so. Subsequently, we will evaluate whether or not we feel fitter compared to how we felt before we began to cycle. We may also engage in 'trial and error' whereby we try a range of regimes before we arrive at the one we consider most effective. Therefore, our everyday experimentation is about cause and effect, determining how one thing has an effect on something else (see definition of Causal Relationship in Chapter 3).

Although this type of experimentation has characteristics of true experiments because we are looking at cause and effect, they cannot be classified as such because they are missing the element of control. In research, there are three factors that are fundamental to a good experiment:

- an intervention
- control
- randomisation.

Intervention

In an experiment there is always an intervention because the researcher is examining the impact of one thing on another. Therefore, without an intervention, there is no experiment. In this type of research design, researchers actively introduce the intervention, which is most commonly described as the independent variable. They then test or measure the effect on the dependent variable. The statement of the relationship between these two variables is referred to as a hypothesis (see definition of Hypothesis in Chapter 3).

Data are collected using tests or measures that are designed to assess the impact of the independent on the dependent variable. It is fundamental that the effect of the intervention can be tested or measured. For example, if researchers want to investigate whether cycling improves fitness they will decide in advance what exact criteria will be used for determining improved fitness. It may be that the researcher wants to focus on aerobic rather than muscular fitness and will therefore use tests that are appropriate to this outcome. Fitness levels will be measured before the introduction of the intervention (cycling) and then again at specified intervals or after a determined period of time. The results are analysed statistically to decide if there is a difference in fitness levels. This would be described as a simple 'before-and-after' study (pre-/post-test) (see Figure 5.1).

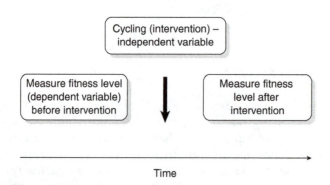

Figure 5.1   A simple experiment

Identify the independent and dependent variables in the list below:

1. A broken leg results in pain.
2. Heart rate increases with exercise.
3. Self-monitoring of blood glucose levels every day leads to better glycaemic control.
4. Practising improves performance.
5. Attendance rate at lectures impacts on examination success.
6. Speed kills.
7. Over-eating causes weight gain.
8. Bacteria cause infections.
9. Skin-to-skin contact between mother and baby after birth promotes bonding.
10. Smoking cigarettes causes chronic obstructive pulmonary disease.

The answers appear at the end of the chapter.

ACTIVITY 5.1

Control

A key feature of the experiment is to ensure with as much certainty as possible that the intervention is responsible for the effect or outcome. In order to do this, the researcher must 'control' for other factors that might lead to uncertainty about the result or outcome.

One of the main strategies adopted to achieve control is the use of two groups where one receives the intervention and the other does not. The group receiving the intervention is known as the 'experimental' group and the other the 'control' group. In healthcare research, it is unlikely that patients receive 'no care'. Therefore, it is usually the case that the experimental group receives the intervention and the control group has the usual, standard or normal care. There can be variations in the number of groups depending on whether there is more than one intervention being tested. All variations where more than one group is used are known as a between-subject or parallel group design (Parahoo, 2006).

Typically, when there are two groups in a study, researchers will attempt to ensure the composition of both groups is similar (homogenous). In practice, this means attempting to guarantee the sample for the study has the same characteristics as the target population. When this is achieved, as far as is possible, the sample is said to be representative of the population and therefore the findings can be said to apply to them (generalisation). This is achieved by drawing the two groups from the same population. The researcher will firstly identify the population of interest for the study. It could be that in our fitness study the researcher wants to focus only on women over the age of 50 and it is from this population that the sample will be drawn. By defining the selection criteria in advance the chances of the intervention and control groups being homogenous are improved.

Participants' characteristics that are controlled for will vary depending on the research question but simple examples include age, gender or illness profile. By doing this, the researcher can say that these factors, known as extraneous variables were controlled and therefore could not account for any differences between the experimental and control group. As a result, the researcher can be more confident that the results arise from the intervention.

No matter how much effort researchers put into ensuring the control and experimental group have the same key characteristics, there is always the potential for differences between them to impact on the study results. Sometimes, therefore, researchers will have only one group in the study that function as both control and experimental group. Essentially, the participants act as their own controls. For example, in a study with 40 participants, 20 can receive the intervention and 20 the usual care after which they swap over. This is known as a crossover or within-subject design (Parahoo, 2006).

ACTIVITY 5.2

Consider an experiment where you wanted to study the effects of cycling on fitness levels. Think of as many factors as you can that might also have an effect on fitness levels.
   Think of how you might 'control' these factors.

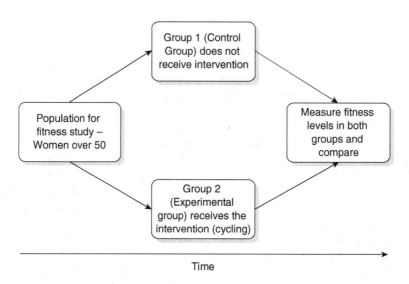

Figure 5.2   An experimental design (with two groups)

Randomisation

The third feature of a good experiment is randomisation where all participants in a study are randomly allocated to either the experimental or control group. Randomisation is another form of control and it has two purposes. Firstly, even when efforts are made to ensure the experimental and control groups are evenly matched for visible variables (e.g. age, gender, weight) there may be others such as attitude, health beliefs, etc. that are not known but which may influence the results of the study. Randomisation is the best means of ensuring there is an equal distribution between the two groups of these unknown variables.

   The sampling strategy adopted to achieve randomisation is known as probability sampling, which is considered the most rigorous because it gives every member of the target population the opportunity to be part of the study. There are several types of probability sampling that include simple, stratified, systematic, cluster and multi-stage (see Chapter 6 for further detail). In our fitness example, all women over the age of 50 would be eligible for the fitness study. The sample would be drawn from this population and then they are randomly allocated to either the experimental or control group (see Figure 5.2).

Secondly, randomisation is a strategy for reducing the potential for what is known as selection bias on the part of the researcher. For instance, if the researcher selected participants to receive the intervention because they thought they might benefit most from it. In our fitness example, the researcher may know that women who are more motivated to become fit are more likely to engage with the intervention.

There are a number of ways to undertake randomisation that can vary from tossing a coin, to picking names/numbers from a hat or using more complex strategies involving computer packages. Sometimes, what is known as 'blind' allocation is undertaken and can be single- or double-blind. In a single-blind trial either the researcher(s) or the participants are unaware of the group to which they have been allocated while in a double-blind study, neither the researcher(s) nor participants know.

Application of Experimental Designs in Healthcare Research

The application of the experimental method in healthcare research is the randomised controlled trial (RCT), which is considered the gold standard for studying the effectiveness of clinical interventions such as new treatments or drugs. The reason for this is that an RCT has all the elements of a good experiment (intervention, control, randomisation).

RCTs are not the only type of experiment undertaken in healthcare and you will frequently encounter studies that are labelled quasi-experimental. These studies of which there are several variations tend to be undertaken in the natural setting or 'in the field'. They are similar to a true experiment in that the manipulation of an intervention is always present but the other two criteria of control and randomisation may be missing (Newell & Burnard, 2011). For example, it is often the case that researchers want to test the effect of an independent variable on participants who are already members of a previously formed group such as patients on a particular ward. In these situations, the researcher cannot randomly assign participants to either the intervention or control groups. Therefore, the sampling strategy used is non-probability which includes convenience or purposive sampling (see Chapter 6).

In addition, researchers may not be able to exert control over the characteristics of the population and sample. What this means is the results of the study may be affected by factors related to the composition of the groups and the natural environment in which it is being undertaken and are referred to as 'threats to validity'. For example, if a researcher wanted to measure the performance of students following the introduction of an innovative learning method, there may be differences in the composition of the experimental group and comparison groups such as age profile and gender distribution that impact on the findings.

As a result the researcher will not be able to say with confidence that the results are due to the intervention. Thus, outcomes in quasi-experimental designs are less reliable than a true experiment and cannot establish cause and effect. Nonetheless, they are still valuable as they can indicate strong links.

Non-experimental Designs (Numerical Data)

Research in health or social care is not limited to experiments because we are not always testing the effectiveness of an intervention. There are many situations where describing the phenomena of interest or observing and/or examining relationships between variables is important to understanding or gaining insight but without establishing cause and effect. Also, and as stated earlier, there are situations where it would be unethical to conduct an experiment such as withholding a treatment that is known to be beneficial. Collectively, the research designs adopted in these situations are known as non-experimental or observational in the medical literature and the essential difference is that there is no manipulation of the independent variable (intervention). Therefore, if a researcher does not or cannot manipulate the independent variable the research study is classed as non-experimental. For example, human characteristics such as gender, age, illness state, ethnicity, etc. that are the focus of research cannot be manipulated experimentally. Non-experimental designs are broadly classified as descriptive/observational, correlational and causal comparative (see Table 5.2).

5.1 Thoughts/Tips

Studies that gather 'narrative' (word) data are also referred to as non-experimental. This is a broad classification and should not be confused with the non-experimental designs in this section that are focussed on studies that gather 'numerical' data that can be subjected to some form of statistical analysis.

Table 5.2   Classification of non-experimental research

Descriptive/ Observational	Studies that describe a phenomenon and its statistical nature, e.g. frequencies, averages, percentages
Correlational Designs	Correlational designs can study the relationship between one variable and another by examining differences in the dependent variable in two groups or examine the relationship between two or more variables in one group. These can describe a relationship, predict a relationship or investigate performance on several variables
Causal comparative/ ex-post-facto	Causal-comparative designs study the relationship between the independent and dependent variables where it is not possible or unethical to manipulate the independent variable

Descriptive/Observational Designs

Descriptive/observational research broadly focuses on observing or describing a phenomenon to provide a precise account of its existence or nature, its prevalence and/or distribution. The key features of this type of research design are large sample sizes and the use of descriptive statistics (see Chapter 10) to analyse the data (Newell

& Burnard, 2011). These can range from large epidemiological studies that might examine the prevalence (cross-sectional study) of a disease or behaviour at one point in time to smaller scale description within a specific population (e.g. cohort study).

Correlational Designs

Correlational research has a different focus in that it can measure or test the relationship between two or more variables. As indicated in Table 5.2, these can be comparative whereby a dependent variable is compared across two groups. In these instances, the independent variable is usually 'categorical' such as gender, learning style, personality type, medication use. For example, performance on a clinical skill (dependent variable) is compared across males and females (independent variable).

Correlational designs can examine the relationship between two or more variables in *one* group. These can include a simple descriptive correlation where two scores are taken from each participant. The scores signify each variable being examined. These are usually taken at one time as past or future performance is not the focus of study. An example of a simple correlational study is determining a possible relationship between success in examinations and motivation to study. Grades in examinations constitute one variable while motivation to study is the other.

Correlational designs can also be 'predictive' where the purpose of the study is to make a forecast about one variable based on another such as overweight (predictor variable) and the risk of developing type 2 diabetes (criterion variable). It is important to remember, however, that even if it is said there is a strong association between the variables, cause and effect cannot be established in correlational research.

Central to correlational studies is the need to visually represent the data that has been collected. This is done using a 'scattergram' (see Figure 5.3). Both scores from each participant are represented by a point on the plot, the scatter of which are subsequently analysed. The closer they are to a straight line the higher the strength of the relationship.

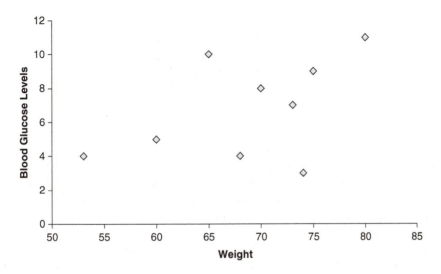

Figure 5.3   Example of a Scattergram

A positive relationship is where a rise in the score of one variable results in a rise in the score of the other while in a negative relationship an increase in one score results in a decrease in the other. An uncorrelated relationship, simply means both variables are independent and not related. Although different criteria may be applied in different contexts for classifying the strength of the relationship, Table 5.3 provides a general rule of thumb. Table 5.4 presents the features and methods in correlational research.

Table 5.3   Classifying the strength of a correlation

Correlation co-efficient	Strength of the Relationship
± 0.29 to 0.00	Weak to none
± 0.30 to 0.69	Moderate
± 0.70 to 1.0	Strong

Table 5.4   Features and methods in correlational research

Purpose	• Examination of the association (relationship) between two or more variables
Paradigm	• Post-positivist
Design	• One point in time
	• Longitudinal as in Predictive; one variable can predict the score on another at a later date (prospective)
Sample	• 30 or greater
	• Heterogenous (different) group to allow for a range of scores
Data collection	• Data are collected on each variable using a measurement tool
Data Analysis	• Scattergram
	○ Relationships are linear, non-linear, uncorrelated
	○ Correlation co-efficient r. Perfect negative correlation (negative linear relationship) represented as −1.0. Perfect positive correlation (positive linear relationship) signified as 1.0. 0.0 indicates no relationship (uncorrelated)
	• Regression/multiple regression – determining if the value of one variable can predict the value of another

Causal-comparative Designs/Ex-post-facto

The third type of non-experimental design in this section are causal-comparative designs. Of the non-experimental designs presented in this section, they are the closest to an experiment. They are used when the research question is causal but it is not possible to manipulate the independent variable. Thus, the essential criterion of manipulation present in experimental and quasi-experimental designs is missing. This applies primarily to people's characteristics such as gender, age, weight, ethnicity, occupation, illness status. For this reason they are also known as ex-post-facto designs because the researcher comes to the situation after the fact has occurred. For example, if researchers are examining the impact of marriage on the health status of a group of people, they cannot manipulate marital status for the purpose of the study. In some situations it would be possible theoretically to manipulate the independent variable but it would be unethical to do so. For instance, in a study investigating recreational drug use, it would be unethical to ask a group of people to take illegal drugs in order to study their impact.

An important point regarding causal-comparative designs is that although the research question is causal, the degree of certainty in respect of claiming the independent variable accounts for the effect on the dependent variable is much smaller than in an experimental study. This is because there may be other extraneous, influencing or confounding variables that may also account for the effect. To illustrate this point let us return to the marital status example. Koball et al. (2010) claim research in this area demonstrates that married people enjoy better physical and mental health than those who are not married. While there may well be an association, being married and better health is not a causal relationship. There are other factors that could impact on the relationship such as the claim that healthy people are more likely to marry and less likely to divorce (Schoenborn, 2004).

Application of Non-experimental Designs in Healthcare Research

The application of non-experimental research that gathers numerical data is primarily through the use of a survey. In many publications, surveys are classified as a research design and considerable time is devoted to discussing their characteristics. Strictly speaking, however, surveys represent a data collection method and for the purposes of this book, are not treated as separate from or independent of the three types of non-experimental research.

Types of Survey

Surveys are a particularly useful means of collecting data because of their versatility. They can be used to simply describe a situation as it exists as in a descriptive survey or can address more complex issues such as associations or comparisons as in correlational and comparative research. McKenna et al. (2010) classify surveys according to the types of non-experimental research discussed above, that is, descriptive, correlational and comparative surveys.

Surveys are further classified according to a time dimension. They can be taken in the present (snap-shot) as in the prevalence (cross-sectional) studies referred to earlier. They can also be retrospective, where information from the past is gathered in an attempt to explain what is happening currently or prospective, where information is gathered into the future.

Retrospective studies are usually undertaken using what are known as 'case-control' approach. 'Cases' such as a group of individuals with a particular outcome, for example, illness/disease are identified and compared with a 'control' group who do not have the identified outcome. Researchers retrospectively examine exposure to risk factor(s) for this illness and undertake a comparison between the cases and the control groups.

Cohort studies, on the other hand, involve observing and recording the development of a specific group of individuals from a defined point in time. They are more commonly prospective but they can be retrospective. Retrospective cohort studies, sometimes referred to as historical cohort studies, use data collected in the past to identify a population and their exposure to an identified risk factor(s). The current disease status (disease/no disease) is then determined for the exposed and non-exposed participants. An important differentiating factor between case-control and retrospective cohort studies is that in the former the outcome (disease status) is measured *before* the exposure to risk factors is examined while in the latter the outcome is measured *after* the exposure (see Figure 5.4).

Prospective studies, observe for the development of an outcome, for example, illness/disease into the future. They are usually longitudinal and data are collected on a number of occasions. An example of a significant international, prospective study is the Framingham study, which began in 1948 with residents of Framingham, Massachusetts who, at the start of the study, had not had a heart attack or stroke or developed overt symptoms of cardiovascular disease. The original purpose was

Case-control study

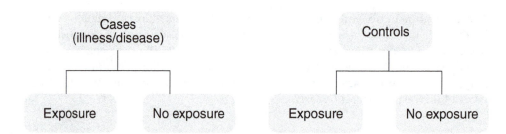

Retrospective Cohort Study

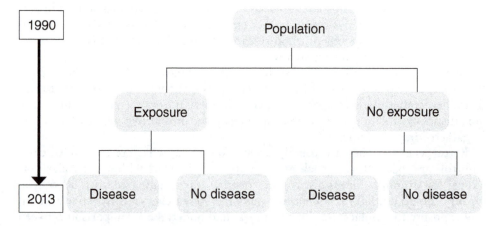

Figure 5.4   Case-control vs Cohort Study

to identify common factors that contribute to cardiovascular disease and exposures included blood pressure, body weight, diabetes, smoking, exercise, etc. Every two years risk factors and the development of cardiovascular disease were measured. The study is ongoing and is now in its third generation of participants and has led to the identification of major CVD risk factors.

Sources of Data in Surveys

Sources of data in surveys are most commonly self-administered questionnaires or structured interviews (Coughlan et al., 2009) but structured observations (non-participant) and secondary data sources such as patient or public records are also used (McKenna et al., 2010). Further detail on these data collection tools is outlined in Chapter 9.

Non-experimental Designs (Narrative/Words)

All studies that do not meet the requirements of an experiment can technically be classed as non-experimental. In this section, we are addressing non-experimental designs that collect narrative (words). Generally speaking studies that collect narrative are classified under the broad term of 'qualitative' research.

The paradigm stance of those who undertake research that is classed as qualitative is essentially different from those who undertake quantitative research and you may see reference to paradigms that include interpretive/constructivist, and critical/transformative/participatory/advocacy among others. Although these paradigms diverge in terms of their overall purpose and outcome they do share broad characteristics about approaches to undertaking research that essentially differ to the positivist or post-positivist stance of those undertaking quantitative research.

One of the fundamental characteristics of qualitative research methodologies is that they seek to interpret and understand human experience from the perspective of the person experiencing it. They are not looking for causal relationships but are seeking to uncover meaning from the perspective of the participant in the study (the *emic* perspective). There is a recognition that each person's truth may be different but both have equal validity.

The researcher does not stand apart but rather engages with the participant and is subsequently fundamental to the interpretation of the data. Thus, the language of qualitative research is different. In using the term 'participants' as opposed to 'subjects', there is a desire to move to partnership in the relationship between the researcher and those involved in the study. Many qualitative research studies are about 'researching with'. As a result, sampling is what is referred to as non-probability sampling. Most frequently, purposive sampling is used but other types include snowball and convenience sampling. For further details on sampling techniques see Chapter 6.

There is a recognition also that human experience cannot be separated from the context in which it happens and the qualitative researcher acknowledges and is sensitive to the context of the lives of those in the study. In addition, qualitative researchers commit to immersing themselves in the world of those with whom they are engaging. In order to achieve this, a variety of data collection methods are employed that include interviewing, observation and examination of personal documents and other printed materials. Chapter 9 discusses these in more detail. In some studies, more than one approach may be used and procedures may be revised as the data collection proceeds.

Participants describe their experiences and they are analysed and interpreted by the researcher and in some cases in partnership with the participants. Moreover, because of the prominence of description of human experiences, there is an emphasis on what is termed 'thick description'. This is more than a superficial description of what is happening in any given situation and involves in-depth exploration of the phenomena being studied.

Data analysis in qualitative research methodologies centres primarily on interpreting the data in order to make sense of it. The process of undertaking data analysis usually involves adopting a systematic approach through the use of an identified framework for analysis (see Chapter 10). The type of framework and the process of analysis varies depending on the desired outcome of the study.

A further feature of qualitative methodologies is the fundamental need to establish trust in the relationship between the researcher and participants. It is expected that researchers adopt a non-judgemental attitude in their approach to the study. This can be difficult to achieve at times as researchers often come to the research question with pre-conceived views on the topic. However, if the findings of the study are to truly reflect the experiences of those who are participating in the study then these pre-conceptions must not influence what data are collected and how they are analysed.

One of the ways in which qualitative researchers attempt to ensure their assumptions do not overly influence how they approach their studies is to undertake critical reflection. This usually involves undertaking a deliberate and explicit reflection on their involvement in the study. This may involve documenting pre-conceptions or assumptions as well as detailing thoughts, feelings and responses to the research and the participants in the study.

The place of theory in qualitative research has been a source of some confusion particularly for novice researchers. Most research texts refer to qualitative methodologies as being theory-generating which is an inductive approach (see Chapter 1) to knowledge generation. This has led some to interpret this to mean that in undertaking a qualitative research study there is no need for reference to or inclusion of theory at the beginning of the study. However, unless researchers are undertaking studies that are explicitly aimed at developing theory, such as Grounded Theory, there is a need to include a theoretical rationale in the study. Creswell (2009) refers to it as a general orienting lens through which the research can be seen. This is often done during the review of the literature where existing theories or concepts on the topic are explored following which the researcher may locate his/her study within a particular framework.

If an existing theory is used to frame the study it is referred to as a 'theoretical' framework whereas if the framework draws on a number of concepts from various theories and research findings, located in the literature, then it is known as a conceptual framework (Parahoo, 2006). See Table 5.5 for examples of theoretical/conceptual frameworks used in qualitative descriptive studies.

Whatever the chosen framework, its use should be explicit throughout the study and should be discussed subsequently in light of the findings. Failure to do so could lead to a sense that the study lacks focus and direction. For example, in Sword et al.'s (2012) qualitative descriptive study, Donabedian's structure, process, outcome model was used as a conceptual framework for exploring women's perspectives on quality pre-natal care. The semi-structured interview guide was informed by the model and addressed questions related to the attributes of the pre-natal healthcare setting (structure), clinical and interpersonal care processes (process) and patient satisfaction (outcomes) (Sword et al., 2012). Subsequently, in the final phase of analysis the emergent themes were assigned to the categories of Donabedian's model, which in turn provided the structure for the discussion of the findings.

If a researcher does not draw on theories, concepts and previous research findings it could be assumed that he/she knows all there is to know about the topic with the result that subsequent findings could be construed as biased. Furthermore, where a theoretical orientation is not mentioned the researcher does little to advance the development of knowledge within a discipline. What this means is that 'atheoretical' studies can only be taken in isolation and they do not add in any way to what is known.

This brief outline of the broad characteristics of non-experimental (narrative) research is not definitive but gives a general picture for the purposes of delineating it from research that is non-experimental and quantitative in nature. The following section focuses on outlining the major qualitative methodologies (see the box below), but a detailed discussion of all of the possible approaches and designs is beyond the scope of this text. Therefore, the reader should access more advanced texts for an in-depth discussion of these methodologies and designs.

Major Qualitative Methodologies

- Qualitative Descriptive Studies
- Grounded Theory
- Phenomenology
- Ethnography
- Narrative
- Action Research
- Case Study

Qualitative Descriptive Studies

According to an editorial by Annells (2007) qualitative description could be considered to be the primary methodology among nurse researchers despite the fact that many research books do not make specific reference to it. There is a view that descriptive research is seen as the simplest form of research and nurses, in an effort to be seen as being methodologically and epistemologically (knowledge) credible, have adopted more sophisticated designs such as phenomenology, grounded theory, ethnography, narrative, etc. (Sandelowski, 2000). The implication is that these methodologies are more scientific and less subject to criticism in terms of the knowledge they produce, which has resulted in a form of demoting of qualitative description. As a possible consequence of its standing, the use and knowledge of qualitative description in healthcare is limited (Neergaard et al., 2009).

The overall purpose of a qualitative descriptive study is to describe or explore a phenomenon, problem or issue and can encompass a broad range of questions relating to people's experiences, knowledge, attitudes, feelings, perceptions and/or views. It is suitable for 'why', 'what', 'where' and 'how', questions. For example, Williams et al. (2008) explored health professionals' and consumers' perspectives on adherence to multiple prescribed medications in diabetic kidney disease while Skårderud (2007) examined the concept of shame and its sub-types in people with a diagnosis of anorexia nervosa.

Qualitative descriptive studies are not guided by a particular philosophical or theoretical orientation in the same way as, for instance, ethnography or grounded theory (see discussion below). This is not meant to imply that qualitative descriptive studies do not have any theoretical underpinning or orientation but that they are more flexible philosophically and theoretically. Because of the questions posed (why, what, where and how), studies of this nature often fall within the interpretivist paradigm (see the box above, p. 60).

 As indicated above, it is important that researchers using qualitative description have some theoretical or conceptual framework from which they approach their studies. This is often done through engagement with the literature. Examples of qualitative descriptive studies that have explicated their theoretical/conceptual framework can be seen in Table 5.5. It is worth noting that in these studies the chosen framework is not always an existing theory but can include models such as that used by Williams et al. (2008) and Sword et al. (2012) or as in the case of the Coenen et al. (2011) study, a framework devised by the World Health Organization (WHO). Features and methods that may be used in qualitative descriptive studies are outlined in Table 5.6.

Table 5.5   Examples of theoretical/conceptual frameworks adopted in qualitative descriptive studies

Author	Title	Theoretical/Conceptual Framework
Williams et al. (2008)	Adherence to multiple prescribed medications in diabetic kidney disease: A qualitative study of consumers' and health professionals' perspectives.	Model of Medication Adherence in Hypertensive Patients (Johnson, 2002).
Coenen et al. (2011)	Functioning and disability in multiple sclerosis from the patient perspective	International Classification of Functioning, Disability and Health framework (ICF) (World Health Organization, 2001)
Rossman et al. (2012)	Healthcare providers' perspectives of breast feeding peer counsellors in the neonatal intensive care unit	Diffusion of Innovations Theory (Rogers, 2003)
Sword et al. (2012)	Women's and care providers' perspectives of quality pre-natal care: a qualitative, descriptive study	Systems-based model of Quality Healthcare – (Structure, process, outcome) (Donabedian, 1988)

Table 5.6   Features and methods in qualitative descriptive studies

Purpose	Describe/explore a phenomenon, problem or issue. It is suitable for 'why', 'what', 'where' and 'how', questions
Paradigm	Interpretivist (most commonly)
Sampling	Non-probability
Data collection	Commonly
	• Once off, face-to-face, semi-structured interviews (individual or groups)
	Rarely
	• In-depth, unstructured interviews with follow-up interviews
Data analysis	Interpreted and *reduced* by creating themes using generic data analysis framework, e.g. Creswell (2009)

Grounded Theory Studies

The term grounded theory refers to the notion that the theory, which is an outcome of the study, is 'grounded' in the data. In 1967, two social science researchers, Glaser and Strauss, published a book entitled *The Discovery of Grounded Theory* that represented the beginning of the emergence of grounded theory as a significant research methodology in healthcare. Glaser and Strauss investigated hospital staff's interactions with dying patients and described how they developed a theory from their data. This grounded theory methodology refers to a systematic set of procedures that are used to develop substantive theories about psychosocial phenomena (Draucker et al., 2007: 1137). The methodology has since evolved with rigorous debate about aspects of the approach by its various proponents. As a result, there are now a number of versions from which researchers can choose.

Although there are similarities with other qualitative research methodologies, there are important distinctions in how a grounded theory study is undertaken if it is to be classed as such. It is often the case that grounded theory is used in circumstances where theories do not already exist. Fundamental to any grounded theory study is that the researcher does not begin with preconceptions about what is happening in the situation under study. That is not to say that researchers do not have some ideas about what is happening but these must not influence the direction and focus of the study. Thus, the researcher does not adopt a theory or a particular theoretical stance at the beginning of the study. There is no theoretical framework and grounded theory studies are referred to as 'truly inductive' (Ross, 2012: 92).

In some approaches such as in classic grounded theory, Glaser and Strauss (1967) advised *against* undertaking a literature review at early stages in the research process. Although this has been the subject of considerable debate also, the rationale for not engaging with the literature at the outset is seen as part of the process of trying to ensure that data collection, analysis and the development of theory are not influenced by existing theoretical perspectives. In this way, categories that would constitute the 'new' theory would emerge naturally during data analysis (Dunne, 2011).

Other key features of grounded theory studies are 'theoretical sampling' and 'constant comparison'. Theoretical sampling refers to the approach to identifying who should be part of the study (see Chapter 6). Initially, the researcher identifies individuals or groups who know about the area of study. The data collected are then analysed and concepts/codes identified. These concepts are explored in subsequent waves of data collection by engaging with various participants or in various settings. Therefore, theoretical sampling differs from other types of sampling in that it is not definitively planned at the beginning of the study but is directed by the emerging concepts and theory. Data collection continues until data saturation occurs, which simply stated means when there are no new data emerging.

The method of data analysis in grounded theory known as constant comparison goes hand in hand with theoretical sampling. The researcher decides what data will be collected next on the basis of the theoretical ideas emerging from previous stages. New data, as they are collected are then compared with what was previously collected. This process of constantly comparing progresses until no more new information is emerging. An important point in the process is that as concepts within the emerging theory become evident, the literature, which is viewed as more data, is sourced in order to achieve a broader understanding. Features and methods that may be used in grounded theory studies are presented in Table 5.7.

Table 5.7   Features and methods in grounded theory studies

Purpose	Generation of substantive theories about psychosocial phenomena that is grounded in the data
Paradigm	Most commonly constructionism but can also be positivist
Sampling	Theoretical Sampling
Data collection	• Interviewing (unstructured or semi-structured) • Observation • Document analysis
Data analysis	• Data collection and data analysis undertaken simultaneously • Constant comparison

Phenomenology

Before presenting the tenets of phenomenology as a basis for conducting research in healthcare, it is important to note that there has been considerable debate within the literature about how it is interpreted and used as a basis for research. This is because phenomenology is primarily a philosophy with a number of styles, a number of schools and a large number of phenomenologists rather than a scientific research method. Its attraction in healthcare has been associated with the development of means to study and understand individuals' subjective experiences. However, in the translation from philosophy to a basis for undertaking research competing views exist about what constitutes phenomenological research and how it should be conducted. Moreover, the language of phenomenology is difficult and complex and if the work of the original philosophers is sourced it becomes almost unfathomable. In addition, there has been some criticism about how studies that claim to be phenomenological fail to adhere to the philosophical concepts or do not outline clearly how these concepts impacted on the conduct of the study (Norlyk & Harder, 2010). All of this can be quite confusing for those who are new to research particularly where they are required to determine if a study claiming to be phenomenological meets the criteria to be deemed as such.

In healthcare research, studies have been conducted that can be aligned with three major streams of phenomenology, namely descriptive, interpretive and existential. The former two have been the most dominant within nursing and midwifery research and are associated with two German philosophers, Edmund Husserl and Martin Heidegger. Differences between these philosophies have implications for any researcher who is undertaking a phenomenological study. Therefore, it is essential that researchers explain which phenomenological philosophy is underpinning their research and delineate how it influenced the subsequent steps of the research process.

Fundamental to any study that claims to be phenomenological is the concept of 'life-world' or 'lived experience'. The term was coined by Husserl who has been credited with the birth of modern phenomenology. In general, the aim is to describe and interpret human experience from the perspective of those experiencing it. The starting point is the life-world and includes the 'everyday world of common experiences' (Holloway & Wheeler, 2010: 219). Thus, life-world experiences such as 'living with diabetes', 'the experience of chronic fatigue', 'caring for a family member with dementia' are chosen and studied in depth.

In Husserlian phenomenology, the focus is on description of the experience (descriptive phenomenology) in order to get at its 'essence' (true meaning) or 'essential structure'. Husserl believed that in 'getting at' the essence of a phenomenon it was possible to identify common themes that relate to each other. However, in order to do so, previous understandings (natural attitude) of the phenomenon must be 'bracketed'. This bracketing, also referred to as phenomenological reduction, reduces the risk of contamination of the participants' descriptions of their experiences. What is most important is the description of the 'phenomenon' itself not the researcher's interpretation of it. The researcher does not make judgements because the emphasis is describing the participants' experience not explaining it. Objectivity in terms of the researcher's position is a distinguishing feature of Husserlian phenomenology (Dowling & Cooney, 2012).

Although there are other differences between Husserl and Heidegger it is on this point that they essentially digress. Heidegger argued that we cannot detach ourselves from the world in which we live or our interpretation of it. Therefore, the focus in Heideggarian (interpretive) phenomenology and in the work of hermeneutic philosophers such as Gadamer and Ricoeur, who were influenced by Heidegger, is on interpretation and understanding rather than description. This, Heidegger argued, is because it is not possible to describe the essence of a phenomenon without interpreting it in the context of our own understanding. Thus, bracketing is not possible. It is evident then that adopting either a Husserlian or Heideggerian approach has fundamental implications for the conduct of a phenomenological study.

In a Husserlian-based study the researcher should outline clearly the phenomenon he/she is addressing, the strategies being adopted to address bracketing and the means by which they have arrived at the essence of the experience. In a Heideggerian-based study, it is also important to detail the experience being investigated but the researcher should describe how his/her pre-understanding or pre-conceptions have been integrated into the research findings (rather than bracketed). The features and methods that may be used in phenomenological studies are presented in Table 5.8.

Table 5.8   Features and methods in phenomenological studies

Purpose	• Description of and experience (descriptive phenomenology) in order to get at its 'essence' • Interpretation to arrive at an understanding of 'what it means' to experience
Paradigm	Interpretivist
Sampling	Purposive
Data collection	• Multiple, individual, in-depth, unstructured interviews • Diary-writing • Observation (Heideggarian) – studying people as they are practically engaged in life
Data analysis	• Description of the essence of the phenomenon (Husserlian) – Colaizzi (1978); Giorgi (1997, 2000a, 2000b, 2006) • Interpretation & Understanding (Heideggarian/ hermeneutic) – Vancouver School, Fleming et al. (2003)

Ethnography

Ethnography is the study of the culture and social structure of groups and has its roots in anthropology. Traditionally, ethnographers studied cultures other than their own by seeking to become accepted within and participating in its life and practices (Robson, 2011). However, modern ethnographers study social relationships across a wide range of groups and often within their own cultural setting. It is an approach commonly used in social and healthcare research.

Ethnographers study cultural groups in order to uncover, describe and interpret the shared communication system, values, beliefs, behaviours and practices that may not be apparent to those who are not part of the group. There are various types of ethnography that have been described by Holloway and Wheeler (2010) as descriptive, critical and autoethnography. In descriptive ethnography, the purpose is to describe the cultural group while critical ethnography is more political and is concerned with factors such as power for the ultimate purpose of change. In autoethnographic studies, the focus is on the experiences of the researcher rather than the experiences of others. Despite their differences, however, they are similar in terms of how the study is conducted.

In ethnographic studies researchers enter and immerse themselves in the setting they wish to study for the purpose of obtaining the subjective view of the members of the group (*emic* or insider view) (see the box below). Usually, such a study is undertaken over a long period of time to facilitate this immersion and to enable the researcher to come to an understanding of the cultural behaviour and norms of the group.

Ethnography has the potential to produce rich data but it is a time-consuming and sometimes arduous undertaking. Not only is it necessary to negotiate entry into the setting but researchers must remain cognisant of their role throughout. In addition, the multiple sources of data and the intensity of data collection in the field is demanding. Moreover, the vastness and complexity of the data requires well-developed analytical skills. The features and methods that may be used in ethnographic studies are outlined in Table 5.9.

Table 5.9   Features and methods in ethnographic studies

Purpose	The study of the culture and social structure of groups to uncover, describe and interpret the groups' shared communication system, values, beliefs, behaviours and practices
Paradigm	• Interpretivist • Critical/transformative/participatory/advocacy
Sampling	Purposive

Data collection	• Researcher is instrument of data collection (becoming a participant)
	• Participant observation (Chapter 9)
	
	  o Direct observation
	  o Interviewing
	
	• Use of pictures, images, symbols

Data analysis	• Write an ethnography (narrative account of the cultural group) – *etic* (outsider's view) • 'Thick description' of the patterns of social and cultural relations

Aspects of Social Setting that Ethnographers Study

- The location or study setting
- The people in the setting
- The activities or actions of individuals and/or the group
- The objects that form part of the setting
- The events that take place
- The timing or sequencing of events
- What people are aiming to do
- The feelings people in the group may have.

(Adapted from Spradley, 1979: 78)

Narrative Research

At the beginning of this section, we stated we were addressing non-experimental designs that collect narrative (words). The introduction now of a methodology called narrative inquiry (research) might cause some confusion. In its broadest sense, narrative can be said to be discourse or anything people might say. However, narrative as a research method adopts a narrower and more technical conception and is defined as spoken or written text that gives an account of something (event(s) and/or action(s)) that are connected (Paley & Eva, 2005; Creswell, 2007).

Narrative research or inquiry is based on the idea that as human beings we come to understanding and give meaning to our lives through story. Although Creswell

(2007) states different fields of study have adopted their own approaches, narrative research has elements of interpretivist and constructivist philosophy. It has long been associated with literary analysis and criticism but has become increasingly accepted as a means of accessing the meaning of patients' suffering and illness in healthcare research. Work such as *The Illness Narratives* by Kleinman (1988) has served to bring to the fore the notion that healthcare professionals can gain valuable insight into the lives and experiences of people in our care. In addition, in telling their stories people can achieve a better understanding of their own experiences.

Narrative research is concerned with asking a research question that is answered by gathering data in the form of stories or accounts. Through analysis and evaluation, the outcome may be a re-storying of the events and/or an identification of themes or patterns. Although there are considerable variations in the approach, Overcash (2003) considers it to be a scientific tool and a process like any other research methodology.

Narrative research is contextual in that it takes place within the lives of the people in the study including time, place, history culture, home, jobs, etc. Clandinin and Connolly (2000: 50) explain this by stating that any narrative inquiry is defined by a three-dimensional space. They have temporal (time) dimensions, they focus on interaction (personal and the social) and they occur in specific places.

Although researchers come to the study with their own 'stories', the participants are empowered in narrative. They tell what they want to tell and choose what it is that is important in the telling. Researchers need to be highly reflexive throughout as they will come to the research with their own story and are not value free (Hardy et al., 2009).

Undertaking narrative research is challenging. From an ethical perspective, researchers undertaking such a study should attend to the notion that institutional ethical approval, which is a requirement, may compromise the notion of truly collaborative and participatory research. Process consent, which involves re-negotiation of consent throughout the study, is essential in a narrative inquiry as it is likely, through negotiation and collaboration, that aspects of the conduct of the study may change.

As mentioned above, narrative research is concerned with the stories as told by the participants in the study. Because of this, there have been criticisms levelled about its anecdotal nature and the difficulty of differentiating fact from fiction. However, in healthcare, it has been argued also that it is this very perspective that adds value. The experience of illness and suffering is highly individual and cannot be accounted for by generalisations.

The extensive data that are gathered in narrative research make analysis complex. Getting at the essence of a person's story, Creswell (2007: 57) states, requires a 'keen eye'. Therefore, being aware of the influence of one's own story and collaboration with the participants is essential. The features and methods that may be used in narrative research studies are outlined in Table 5.10.

Action Research

Action research is an approach to research that involves undertaking research *with* people rather than *on* them. It has been defined by Reason and Bradbury (2008: 4) as

Table 5.10   Features and methods in narrative research studies

Purpose	Gaining insight into the lives and experiences of people through story
Paradigm	Interpretivist or Constructivist
Sampling	Purposive
Data collection	• Researcher is a collaborator/facilitator • Observation • Interviewing • Written journals or diaries • Artefacts, letters, documents
Data analysis	• Re-storying – producing a chronological narrative (beginning, middle and end) (Creswell, 2007)
	And/or
	• Establish the meaning of the story through identification of themes and patterns arising from the data

a participatory process ... it seeks to bring together action and reflection, theory and practice, in participation with others, in the pursuit of practical solutions to issues of pressing concern to people ...

Key features of action research studies include: the participation of those in a specific situation, problem solving related to an issue that is identified as needing development/improvement and identification and enactment of an intervention (change) to achieve the desired outcome. This process is often cited as the action research cycle as represented in Figure 5.5.

Action research has been used extensively in education but in recent years has been adopted more widely in health and social care research. Reason and Bradbury (2008) describe action research as a 'family of practices of inquiry' and suggest there is no one correct way of doing it. The focus can vary from examining one's own practice, the collective practice of others, the development of organisations or even rectifying power imbalances in society for the benefit of ordinary people.

According to Meyer (2010), a useful typology is that of Hart and Bond (1995) who cite four basic types of action research: experimental, organisational, professionalising and empowering. Each type signifies different theoretical perspectives in respect of knowledge and knowledge production. For example, experimental types

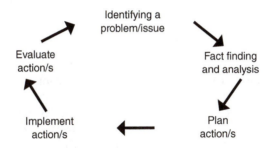

Figure 5.5   Action research cycle

of action research tend to be associated with testing, measuring, controlling and generalising, which is in keeping with positivist or post-positivist paradigms. Conversely, empowering action research focuses on empowering users/practitioners, negotiating outcomes and acknowledging fluidity, which is more in keeping with a critical/participatory/advocacy paradigm. In healthcare, there is an increasing emphasis on the empowering models of action research, which accounts for its classification as a qualitative research approach. However, it is important for readers to bear in mind that not all action research can be classed as such.

In action research, the first stage of the process (see Figure 5.5) is identifying a problem or an issue that needs to change or improve. Subsequently, the researcher works with the participants to identify the research question and membership of the action research group. Prior to planning the change further analysis is undertaken in order to clarify the participants' views on what needs to change. The findings are reported back to the membership and a plan of action is devised. The plan of action includes agreeing the change to be implemented, the timeline for the change, the roles and responsibilities of members of the group and the resources needed (Meyer, 2010; Ross, 2012).

During the implementation phase, monitoring of the change and its effects are undertaken. Interim findings from monitoring the change and its effects often results in re-evaluation and revision of the plan.

Deciding when an action research study has come to an end is difficult but the researcher needs to withdraw from the setting at some point. This may have been determined at the outset by the project time-scale and it is at this point that an evaluation of the implementation of the planned change is undertaken.

Action research is seen as highly relevant for healthcare as it has the potential to generate solutions to problems in practice that are context specific. Moreover, it encourages practitioners in the setting to become involved in devising such solutions resulting in ownership and empowerment. However, there are difficulties that can be encountered. According to its proponents, the strength of action research is its collaborative and participatory nature. Thus, it could be argued that the success of action research projects is dependent on these and when they are not achieved for whatever reason, the project is put at risk.

Action research is complex and can take a considerable amount of time because of the cyclical processes of planning, action, evaluation and amending the plan. In addition, conflict can occur in groups particularly in relation to agreeing problems and solutions and according to Ross (2012) the larger the group, the greater the potential for conflict. The features and methods that may be used in action research studies are outlined in Table 5.11.

Case Study

In case study research the *case* is a unit (an individual, a phenomenon, an activity, a decision, an innovation, a service, a programme), a group or an entity such as a school, a community, a university, a hospital, an organisation. It can involve single or multiple cases and its essential, defining characteristic is that the research undertaken concentrates on the case/s in its own right (Robson, 2011). The cases have clear boundaries and are studied in context because they always occur in a physical and social setting.

Table 5.11   Features and methods in action research studies

Purpose	Problem solving related to an identified issue and enactment of a change to achieve the desired outcome
Paradigm	• Positivist/post-positivist • Critical/participatory/advocacy
Sampling	Purposive

Data collection	• Identifying the problem/issue phase
	  o Questionnaires
	  o Interviews and/or focus groups
	• Implementation phase
	  o Documentary review
	  o Participant observation
	  o Field notes
	  o Diaries and reflective journals
	• Evaluation phase
	  o Audit
	  o Reflection through interviews, focus groups

Data analysis	Varies according to the type of data that have been collected

Case study research is used in a wide range of disciplines (Robson, 2011). It can be qualitative, quantitative or a mixture of both but the qualitative case study is more common in healthcare research (Holloway & Wheeler, 2010). Qualitative case study design is seen as theory generating, rather than theory testing and can be regarded therefore as congruent with interpretivism or constructivism (Ross, 2012).

As indicated above, case studies can vary according to their size but they can also be characterised by their intention. Stake (2005) identified three types, namely: instrumental, collective and intrinsic case studies. Instrumental case studies examine a particular case in order to gain insight into an issue. In collective (or multiple) case studies, several cases are studied jointly. It is an instrumental case extended to study a number of cases. Intrinsic case studies are undertaken to gain a deeper understanding of the case itself.

Undertaking case study is appropriate when there are clearly identifiable and delimited cases that are amenable to in-depth study. The selected cases may be ordinary, accessible or unusual (Creswell, 2007). Sampling can be complex and must be undertaken carefully. There is the potential for attrition (drop-out), which has serious implications for studies that have only one or two participants. If an organisation or institution constitutes the case there is added complexity. For example, if a researcher studying a hospital wished to capture the perspectives of the functioning sub-units (departments) and those that use those departments (professionals, patients) the sampling strategy would be far more complex than if he/she remained at the level of the whole (institution).

Challenges in case study research begin with identifying an appropriate case as there may be more than one that is worthy of study. A decision must also be taken about whether more than one case is included and if so, how many? Creswell (2007) suggests that the researcher will choose no more than four or five cases. It must be recognised, however, that in choosing multiple cases, the researcher may sacrifice depth (Stake, 2005). The features and methods that may be used in case study research are outlined in Table 5.12.

Table 5.12   Features and methods in case study research

Purpose	Identify and study a single or multiple cases in order to gain insight into an issue or gain a deeper understanding of the case itself
Paradigm	• Positivist/post-positivist • Interpretivist • Constructivist
Sampling	Purposive
Data collection	Multiple sources
	• Interviews • Observation (direct and participant) • Documentation • Audio-visual material • Archival records • Artefacts
	(Yin, 2013)
Data analysis	• Analysis can be *holistic* (complete case is presented) or *embedded* (focus on one aspect) • May begin with a description of the case (history, chronology of events, daily activities) • If more than one case, thematic analysis of each (*within-case analysis*) may be undertaken and followed by a thematic analysis across the cases (*cross-case analysis*)

Mixed Method Research

Finally, it is important to mention that you may encounter studies that are referred to as mixed method, triangulation or multi-method research. These are studies that combine or blend methods that are normally associated with different paradigms in one study. Mixed method research emerged because its proponents argue it can provide a more holistic view of a phenomenon, which can lead to greater understanding. For example, a controlled trial can produce statistics that demonstrate the most effective treatment for a patient but it does not tell us if the patient will be willing to take the drug. Therefore, complementing the statistical study with interview data can provide greater insight. In some situations, the data from mixed method studies can offer greater certainty. However, Parahoo (2006) highlights that inconsistent or divergent findings can result in great uncertainty.

Simons and Lathlean (2010: 331) argue that it is important that the two methods adopted in the study must interact and simply using methods in 'tandem' does not constitute mixed methods. Convergence or blending can be sequential whereby the findings from one method can be extended by adopting another (Creswell, 2009). For example, a study could begin with interviews or focus groups and the results are used to inform the development of a survey questionnaire that is subsequently used with a larger sample. Alternatively, a study could begin with a survey questionnaire with the results being subjected to deeper exploration with a small group of individuals. Blending can also occur where methods to collect numerical and narrative data are undertaken concurrently with both sets of data ultimately informing the overall interpretation of the results (Creswell, 2009).

Those that support the use of mixed method argue that it is pragmatic (practical) and the fact that it may cut across research designs and paradigms is less important than providing answers to questions. However, universal agreement on this stance is not evident and there are those who would suggest that mixing methods is not appropriate because paradigms are essentially incompatible.

For further discussion, many research texts devote chapters to mixed method research and since 2007 the *Journal of Mixed Methods Research* has been in publication.

Chapter Summary

This chapter presented an overview of a number of research designs that are used in healthcare research. The chapter began with an outline of the paradigms that most commonly underpin the various research designs used in healthcare. The research designs were broadly classified as experimental, quasi-experimental and non-experimental. The non-experimental designs were divided into those that collect numerical data and those that focus on narrative (words) data. The characteristics of each research design were explained and their relevance to the practical endeavour of undertaking a study outlined. The chapter concluded with a brief introduction to mixed method research.

🗝 Key Points 🗝

- All research designs have certain characteristics that define them and distinguish them from each other.
- Researchers adopt a particular view or stance about how knowledge is developed and these are categorised into a number of paradigms.
- Experimental designs have three fundamental elements: intervention, control and randomisation. The application of the experimental method in healthcare research is the randomised controlled trial (RCT).
- Non-experimental designs are broadly classified as descriptive/observational, correlational and causal comparative.
- The application of non-experimental research that gathers numerical data is primarily through the use of a survey.
- Non-experimental research that collects narrative data is largely aligned with qualitative methodologies.
- Major qualitative methodologies are Qualitative Description, Grounded Theory, Phenomenology, Ethnography, Narrative, Action research and Case study.
- Studies that are referred to as mixed method, triangulation or multi-method research combine or blend methods that are normally associated with different paradigms in one study.

Useful Online Resources

www.socialresearchmethods.net

ANSWERS TO ACTIVITY 5.1

Key: Independent variable (IV); Dependent variable (DV)

1. A broken leg (IV) results in pain (DV).
2. Heart rate (DV) increases with exercise (IV).
3. Self-monitoring of blood glucose levels every day (IV) leads to better glycaemic control (DV).
4. Practising (IV) improves performance (DV).
5. Attendance rate at lectures (IV) impacts on examination success (DV).
6. Speed (IV) kills (DV).
7. Overeating (IV) causes weight gain (DV).
8. Infections (DV) are caused by bacteria (IV).
9. Skin-to-skin contact between mother and baby after birth (IV) promotes bonding (DV).
10. Smoking cigarettes (IV) causes chronic obstructive pulmonary disease (DV).

6

Understanding Sampling and Sampling Size

Introduction

The idea of gathering data about individuals is not a modern concept. The Bible makes reference to Caesar Augustus who lived between 63 B.C. and 23 A.D. undertaking a census of the population (St. Luke's Gospel). Similarly, William the Conqueror was responsible for the 'Domesday Book', a census of the population of his kingdom, which was completed in 1086. Both of these censuses were undertaken for the purpose of taxation, so would have sought to include the total population to ensure everyone paid their dues.

Nowadays, population census is used in situations such as a 'quinquennial' or a 'decennial' census, by which modern states attempt to plan future needs by gathering data such as the gender, age and number of citizens in a country. However, these types of data gathering exercises by their nature are cumbersome, require a major degree of planning, are time consuming, are costly to undertake and necessitate a lot of resources to analyse the data gathered. To ensure accuracy there is also a legal obligation on citizens to participate. For the modern researcher a more user friendly way of selecting individuals from whom to gather data is necessary, rather than attempting to include everyone. Thus, the concept of sampling the population was conceived.

The methods used to select a sample vary, depending on the type of research being undertaken and what the researcher is attempting to achieve. The size of the sample will also vary. Studies that collect numerical data will usually have a bigger sample size than those that collect narrative (words) data. However, researchers are sometimes forced to compromise on their sample size because of issues such as the availability of participants or time constraints on the study. The purpose of this chapter is to introduce the reader to the different approaches used in selecting samples and how different sampling methods are used to support the underlying philosophical principles of the methodology selected.

☑ **Learning Outcomes** ☑

By the end of this chapter you should be able to:

- List the different types of sample
- Identify the different techniques used to select samples
- Differentiate between probability and non-probability sampling methods
- Discuss the importance of sample size.

Populations

A population may be defined as all the components that are deemed to have one or more common characteristics and therefore constitute a group. The characteristics of this group are determined by the researcher and may consist of people, artefacts, incidents or materials depending on the focus of the research. In health science research populations commonly refer to people. However, where other items are used as sources of data, the principles underpinning the identification of populations and samples are similar.

As previously stated a population is all of the individuals or items that share one or more criteria that are predetermined by the researcher. In the case of a 'quinquennial' or a 'decennial' census, this is all the individuals who are resident in the country on one pre-arranged night. In this case, all living individuals in the country meet the criteria and therefore form the target population. Thus, a census of the population is not a sample because all of the individuals in the target population are included in the study.

When undertaking research it is necessary for the researcher to set the sampling criteria that will identify the individuals or items that will be the focus of the study. It is to this group of individuals that the researcher undertaking a quantitatively-based study will attempt to make inferences in relation to the findings. This group is known as the '*target or theoretical population*'. The target population can be a large dispersed group of individuals, which may make accessing them quite difficult, so researchers will sometimes identify an '*accessible or study population*'. This group will be reasonably accessible for the researcher and will be the group from which the sample will be drawn. It is important to note at this stage that the study population should be representative of the target population if inferences to the latter population are to be made (Grove et al., 2013).

Sampling Criteria

When determining the target population the researcher identifies characteristics that help define who fits in the population. These criteria are known as sampling or eligibility criteria (Grove et al., 2013). To specify who has the characteristics of the target population the researcher distinguishes between those who will be part of the population – *Inclusion Criteria* – and those who will be omitted from the population and therefore the study – *Exclusion Criteria*. The criteria for both inclusion and exclusion should be justified by the researcher as these will impact on who is part of the population. In the past, characteristics such as gender, religion and race have been cited as exclusion criteria (Larson, 1994, cited by Grove et al., 2013). While it may be necessary to exclude groups for explicit reasons, generally the principles of inclusivity should apply. Some of the more common exclusion criteria include the inability to read or speak a particular language, as the person may not be able to complete a questionnaire or partake in an interview; under 18 years – due to issues of consent; or non-registration in a particular professional registration body, for example the Chartered Society of Physiotherapists or the Nursing and Midwifery Council.

Selecting a Sample

Due to the fact that most populations are large and unwieldy, it is not usually possible to include everyone in the accessible population in the study. It is then necessary to select a sample from this population. As quantitatively- and qualitatively-based research differ in their research focus, quantitative research focusing on measurable outcomes and generalisation of results to the target population and qualitative research focusing on describing or understanding phenomenon through people's experiences and the development of theories, their approaches to sampling also differ. Some methods of sampling can be seen in Table 6.1.

Table 6.1   Probability and non-probability sampling methods

Probability Sampling	
Simple Random Sample	This is the most straightforward method of achieving a sample that is probably representative of the population. A sample frame with the names of the target population is required and the sample is randomly drawn using manual or computer-based strategies
Systematic Random Sample	Elements are selected at specified intervals from a randomised sampling frame. The first element selected is identified using a table of random numbers
Stratified Random Sample	Used where the target population contains specific groups that need to be identified separately within the sample
Cluster Sampling (Multi-stage Sampling)	Most commonly used where the sample is dispersed over a large geographical area but the researcher needs a probability sample that is clustered into a small number of sites
Non-Probability Sampling	
Convenience (Accidental) Sampling	Individuals who are easily accessible are selected to form a sample, for example people entering or leaving a building. This type of sample is rarely representative
Consecutive Sampling	This is a more comprehensive form of convenience sampling in that members of the accessible population are included in the sample on a 'first come first selected basis'

(Continued)

Table 6.1   (Continued)

Non-Probability Sampling	
Quota Sampling	This is a more complex form of convenience sampling in that the researcher identifies sub-groups within the population and identifies the numbers of individuals in each sub-group that should participate based on the target population. However, participant selection is based on availability
Volunteer Sampling	The researcher uses posters or other forms of media to invite participants who meet certain criteria to participate in the study. This is again a form of convenience sampling
Snowball (Network) Sampling	Used to access individuals from less accessible or closeted populations such as sex-trade workers or gay / lesbian individuals. A member of the group is sought who will access a number of individuals who in turn access others. This again is a convenience method of selecting individuals
Purposive (Judgemental) Sampling	Most common form of sampling used in narrative- (word) based research and is used to select individuals who have experience of the phenomenon being investigated and will therefore most benefit the study
Theoretical (Theory-based) Sampling	Form of sampling used in Grounded Theory to purposively select individuals whose experience and knowledge can advance the theory being developed by the researcher

In research that focuses on numerical data, a sample may be described as a group of individuals, from the target population, who are selected to represent that populace. It is important to attempt to select a sample that is representative of the target population if the researcher wishes to make inferences about the findings in the sample to the target population. This is known 'generalising'. Selecting a sample that is truly representative of the target population is almost impossible. However, there is a way of increasing the likelihood of sample representativeness and this is done through 'probability sampling'. Probability sampling does not guarantee a representative sample; it only offers the 'probability' that the sample will be representative. Similarly, non-probability samples are not guaranteed to be non-representative, but there is a strong chance that they will not be representative of the target population. Examples of where non-representative sampling has led to incorrect conclusions are included in the box below.

In research that gathers narrative (words) data where the aim is to gather in-depth knowledge and information on a phenomenon, the type of sample required is different. Instead of needing a sample that represents the target population, a sample that has experience of the phenomenon is required. The most common method used to select a sample in qualitative research is purposive sampling.

Historical Inaccuracies Using Non-probability Sampling

History demonstrates the problems of attempting to generalise findings that are not representative of the population. During the 1936 US Presidential Elections a poll undertaken by the Literary Digest predicted that Alfred M. Landon would have a landslide victory over the incumbent President Franklin D. Roosevelt to become the next US President. In fact Franklin D. Roosevelt won the election. So where did the Literary Digest Poll go wrong?

The Literary Digest had a previous good record of predicting US presidential elections and had predicted the presidential winner correctly in the previous five elections. In this survey they sampled 10 million Americans (about a quarter of the electoral register) using car registration lists, the subscription list to the magazine, and telephone directories, and had a response rate of over two million participants. The two factors that appear to have caused this incorrect prediction were the non-representative convenience sample and the poor response rate (Squire, 1988). The Literary Digest pollsters selected their sample using a form of convenience sampling, a non-probability sampling method which can be unreliable when attempting to generalise a result to the target population. At the time there were few alternative sampling approaches, and this method had predicted correctly for the Literary Digest Company in the past. However, this poll took place during the Great American Depression, where cars, phones and subscriptions to magazines were luxuries that many of the poor in the populace could not afford and therefore this eliminated them from the sample. As it happened many of the poorer members of society appeared to be supporters of Roosevelt. The second factor that influenced the outcome of this poll was a non-response bias. Polit and Beck (2012) define a non-response bias as the potential difference that could occur to the findings of a study, if the non-responders participated in the research. In the 1936 poll there appears to have been a greater number of Republican supporters in the sample and while those that responded appear to have been in the majority Republican (Squire, 1988), a greater overall response rate may have offered a more accurate result despite the unrepresentativeness of the sample.

While this incorrect election prediction signalled the end for the Literary Digest, other survey groups such as Gallup correctly predicted the outcome of the 1936 election using a new sampling approach that became known as quota sampling. This method of sampling was used with an element of success for a number of American presidential elections.

However, in 1948 history repeated itself when Gallup and other pollsters incorrectly predicted that the incumbent President Harry S. Truman would be defeated by Thomas E. Dewey. An interesting aside to this was that internal issues forced the Chicago Daily Tribune

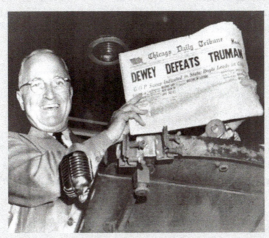

President Harry S. Truman jubilantly holding a copy of the *Chicago Daily Tribune* with the heading that incorrectly predicted his defeat to Thomas E. Dewey in the 1948 Presidential Election

(Continued)

(Continued)

to publish before the election was declared, and faith in the polls contributed to them leading with the headline 'Dewey Defeats Truman' (*Chicago Daily Tribune*, Nov 3rd, 1948, p.1). Quota sampling is a form of convenience sampling in which the researcher attempts to reflect the constituent groups of the target population in a representative manner in the sample. While this approach appears to offer a sample that may be representative, the researcher is free to decide who will be selected to the different groups within the sample which introduces the risk of interviewer bias. Daniel (2012) states that interviewer bias was one of the factors that could be implicated in the quota sampling failing to correctly predict the outcome in this election.

One of the outcomes of this situation was a move toward probability sampling to select individuals to participate in polls (Daniel, 2012). This method was beginning to become established at the time, and correctly predicted the outcome of this election.

The common factor that led to the inaccurate results in both these election polls was the non-representativeness of the samples which led to results with poor external validity (non-generalisability). Probability sampling, which has become accepted as a more dependable sampling method, has a greater likelihood of being representative and therefore a stronger external validity.

Probability Sampling

A probability sample (also known as a random sample) is one whereby all members of the target population have an equal opportunity of being selected to participate in the study and no individual in the target group is excluded from the opportunity of being selected. It is not, as the word random sometimes implies, an unplanned or haphazard approach to sampling, but a deliberate and systematic sampling method. There are a number of different ways of achieving a probability sample. However, they are not easy to select as the researcher has to have a means of accessing all the members of the target population in order to achieve it. The list, through which all members of the target population are accessed, is known as a sample frame.

Simple Random Sample

A simple random sample is the most straightforward method of acquiring a probability sample. A sample frame with the names of the target population is required and depending on the size, the researcher can select the sample by simply placing all the names in a box and drawing out the number required for the sample. Alternatively, for larger samples, numbers can be assigned to names and a computer programme, such as a random number generator, can be used to select the numbers randomly, or they can be selected from a table of random numbers (see the box below).

A Section from a Table of Random Numbers

72176 18103 55169 79954 72002 20582 65358 70469 87149 89509 00209 90404 99457 72570
80583 70361 41047 26792 78466 03395 17635 09697 82447 31405 42194 49043 24330 14939

01911 60767 55248 79253 12317 84120 77772 50103 05409 20830 80210 34361 52228 33869
89848 48579 06028 03405 01178 06316 81916 40170 53665 87202 88638 94332 83868 61672
09865 64623 82780 35686 30941 14622 04126 25498 95452 63937 95836 22530 91785 45906
10971 90472 44682 39304 19819 55799 24028 47121 78545 49201 05329 14182 12872 13827
96205 27937 45416 71964 52261 30781 02955 86558 84750 43994 01760 77800 25734 14969

There is some debate when drawing names or numbers manually, as to whether a name drawn should be replaced before the next name is drawn. Grove et al. (2013) state that re-including that name or number is the more conservative approach, but as a name or number can only be selected once the overall difference in the probability of selection is probably quite small.

Systematic Random Sample

When employing a systematic random sample the researcher uses a systematically derived interval when selecting individuals from a sample frame. The interval is calculated by dividing the sample frame by the proposed sample size. For example, if the sample frame contained 5,000 individuals and the expected sample size was 500 then the interval would be every 10th individual on the sample frame. However, to ensure randomness within the sample, the sample frame should not be in any organised manner, for instance alphabetical. Also, the first individual selected should be chosen randomly such as from a table of random numbers.

Stratified Random Sample

Selecting a stratified random sample requires the researcher to have a greater knowledge of the composition of the target population. This is because the purpose of this sampling method is to categorise the sample into two or more groups or strata that are representative of target population. Strata can be gender, age group, qualifications and so on. Ensuring that these strata samples are selected in proportion to their numbers in the population, helps to further enhance the probability of representativeness. For example, a study exploring the experiences of nursing students in a university might first develop a sample frame of all nursing students in each year of the course and then might take a sample of 20 per cent of the students in each year (Table 6.2). In this scenario the number of students selected for the study is representative of the size of each year. With a simple random sample this outcome could have potentially been very different (Table 6.3). The first year students are clearly under-represented in the sample and the other years are over-represented especially the fourth year students.

In order to perform a stratified random sample the researcher needs to know what strata exist and be able to obtain the information on the numbers in each group. Access to this information is not always easy to obtain and therefore a simple random approach may be more appropriate. In the case of Table 6.2 below, if the information were available the student groups could be further subdivided into their chosen branch of nursing, for example, Adult, Mental Health, Children, Learning Disability, further increasing representativeness.

Table 6.2   Stratified random sample of nursing students

Students per year	Total Population	Sample
1st year students	250	50
2nd year students	210	42
3rd year students	220	44
4th year students	180	36
Total	860	172

Table 6.3   Simple random sample of nursing students

Students per year	Total Population	Sample
1st year students	250	28
2nd year students	210	44
3rd year students	220	48
4th year students	180	52
Total	860	172

Cluster Sample (Multi-stage Sampling)

When data is being gathered using face-to-face interviews or when the population is large and dispersed over a considerable area, it may not be feasible to use simple or stratified random samples to identify a suitable sample. Particularly where face-to-face interviews are being undertaken, it is easier if the researcher can collect data from individuals that are in reasonably close proximity to each other. Cluster sampling, also known as multi-stage sampling is a method of randomly selecting individuals from randomly selected groups. If a national survey of nurses working in Accident and Emergency (A&E) units was to be undertaken in the UK, a researcher might first develop a sampling frame of all of the A&E units in the country and from this randomly select a number of units to participate. Once these A&E units have been selected the researcher then randomly selects individual nurses from those units to be the sample. It is important to note that because all A&E units were included initially all the nurses in those units had an equal opportunity of being selected and none were excluded from being selected and thus the sample is random.

Non-probability Sampling

Non-probability samples by their nature do not aim to be representative of the target population. As such these samples should not be used by researchers who seek to make inferences from their findings to the population. However in some instances, due to time constraints or lack of a sample frame, a non-probability sample may be all that the researcher has available. In such cases the limitations that arise from selecting a non-probability sample should be identified. Researchers using qualitatively-based methodologies use non-probability samples.

Convenience Sample (Accidental Sample)

Convenience samples can be used in all research designs. This non-probability method of sampling selects individuals or items that are conveniently accessible to the researcher. For example, a researcher may select a sample from clients attending a particular clinic. However clients who do not attend that particular clinic may have different characteristics to those in the sample. While this is not an issue when a researcher is not attempting to generalise the findings, from a quantitative perspective it does reduce the likelihood that accurate inferences can be made to the target population.

Convenience sampling can be a reasonably inexpensive and quick way of obtaining a sample, and may in some cases be the only option available. It does, however, have the potential to increase the risk of what is known as sampling bias. Because there is the potential that the researcher can choose who to approach or include, there is a risk of subjectivity in the selection of the sample (Parahoo, 2006). Despite this, convenience sampling is a commonly used method of selecting a sample (Polit & Beck, 2012).

Consecutive Sample

This form of convenience sample involves choosing individuals, who meet the selection criteria, on a 'first come, first selected' basis until the sample size is achieved or the time frame is complete (Polit & Beck, 2012). It is regarded as being potentially less biased than convenience sampling as it removes subjectivity from selection. In the case of sampling periods it is necessary to ensure that they are sufficiently long to reduce the risk of seasonal variables, such as influenza outbreaks, influencing the outcomes.

Quota Sample

This sampling method is a more complex form of convenience sampling. The sample here is selected from the different strata within the target population. It can be considered as a non-probability form of stratified sampling. To undertake quota sampling, the researcher needs an insight into the different strata that comprises the target population. While quota sampling is not as rigid as stratified random samples it does attempt to have the strata that reflect the target population as closely as possible. However, selection of subjects is undertaken using convenience sampling and the option to include or not to include an individual is a decision that can be consciously or unconsciously made by the researcher leading to the risk of sampling bias.

Volunteer Sample

Parahoo (2006) identifies volunteer sampling as possibly the weakest method of selecting a sample. This approach is, to a large degree, self-selection on the part of the participants. This type of sample may be generated as a result of a poster or an announcement seeking volunteers to participate. Self-selectors may offer to participate because they have an interest in the topic, or because they may be sympathetic towards the researcher (who may be doing the research as part of a course) or for any number of reasons. Their eagerness to participate in itself can make these individuals unrepresentative of the population (Parahoo, 2006). Other groups from whom volunteer samples sometimes derive are captive populations. Parahoo (2006) questions if participation of students in a classroom or patients on a hospital ward is truly voluntary and counsels on the ethical issues related to vulnerable groups.

Snowball Sample

Snowball sampling (also known as network or chain sampling) is used when attempting to obtain a sample from what might be described as a difficult to reach population such as sex-workers or other groups whose membership may not be easily accessible. Members of these groups often have a means of networking with each other and so through accessing one member of the group, others can be encouraged to participate in the study. When using this approach the researcher seeks to recruit a single participant, known as a seed, who will then recruit others who in turn become recruiters (Sadler et al., 2010). An example of snowball sampling can be seen in the box below.

Exemplar Snowball Sampling

Advanced maternal age: Delayed childbearing is rarely a conscious choice. A qualitative study of women's views and experiences

The sample for this group was 18 women between the ages of 35 and 50, six who were childless; six who were undergoing fertility treatment and six who were pregnant with their first child. Snowball sampling was used to recruit for the first group.

> Women who were not pregnant or attending for fertility treatment could not be recruited through the maternity services. A 'snowball' sampling strategy was used; the initial participant recruited to this group was known to one of the researchers and identified a further potential participant who was likely to be information rich, who subsequently identified another potential participant and so on.
>
> (Cooke et al., 2012: 32)

Snowball sampling can be used in quantitatively- or qualitatively-based research to recruit individuals to a study. However, from the quantitatively-based perspective it is a non-probability sample as those recruited to the study are selected as they are known to other members of the sample. This in itself can lead to a bias as the sample may be very homogenous and others with diverse views may not have been recruited.

Purposive Sample

This non-probability method of sampling is the most commonly used in qualitatively-based methodologies such as phenomenology and grounded theory. It is also known as judgemental or purposeful sampling and it involves the researcher selecting individuals to participate on the basis that they can provide a particular insight into the phenomenon being studied, or that they have an extensive knowledge and/

or experience of the phenomenon in question (Grove et al., 2013). Despite rationalising why particular participants should be included and criteria to identify those with knowledge or experience of the phenomenon, participant selection remains subjectively linked to the researcher's beliefs.

Theoretical Sample

This is a form of sampling that is used in grounded theory to select groups of participants who can add to theory development. Initially, samples in grounded theory research may be convenience or purposive but as a theory evolves groups of individuals whose particular experiences can help to support or refute the theory are selected to refine and develop a substantive theory.

Sample Size

A common question asked is 'How big should my sample size be?' The answer to this will depend first on whether the study is collecting numerical or narrative data. In a study that is collecting numerical data, the simple answer is the bigger the sample the better. Larger sample sizes tend to reduce the risk of what are known as Type II Sampling Errors. A Type II Sampling Error occurs when there is a failure to reject the null hypothesis and demonstrate significance in a statistical test. Grove et al. (2013) recommend that as a rule of thumb a researcher should have a minimum of thirty participants for each variable in the study. So if three variables are being studied then ninety participants would be required. The sample would then need to be large enough to allow for non-responders and still achieve the required participant numbers.

Another way to determine an adequate sample size and avoid a Type II Sampling Error is through the use of power analysis. Power analysis is a statistical calculation that includes the power level, the level of significance, the effect size and the sample size. The power level is an indicator of the probability of avoiding a Type II error, and is usually set at 0.8. This means that there is an 80 per cent probability of overcoming a Type II error (Coughlan et al., 2009). The level of significance refers to the probability of the findings occurring by coincidence rather than design. In the Health Sciences significance is most commonly set at ≤0.05 per cent, which means the probability of this result occurring by accident is less than or equal to five in a hundred. Effect size relates to the strength of the relationship between the variables. A strong relationship usually requires a smaller sample size to demonstrate it exists while weaker relationships require larger sample sizes (Polit & Beck, 2014). As the sample size is the final determinant in a power analysis, when the other factors are set the analysis will determine the minimum number of participants required.

In narrative-based research the focus is on the quality of the data collected rather than on attempting to undertake statistics or to generalise to the target population. Consequently, the sample size in these types of samples are smaller. In determining sample size, the factors that need to be considered are the richness and depth of the information that is being gathered and data saturation. One of the main reasons for a lack of depth or richness in describing the phenomenon being explored is that the sample size is too small. This is particularly the case where the theme being explored is broad and more participants are required to adequately explore the phenomenon. A lack of richness and depth tends to undermine the credibility of the findings (Polit & Beck, 2014).

Data saturation, for many qualitative researchers, is an aspiration, rather than an achievable outcome. It is said to have been achieved when no new themes on the phenomenon are emerging from participants' descriptions and what is being gathered echoes previous data. Data saturation is not easy to achieve and in fact Morse (1989), cited by Streubert and Carpenter (2011), states that it is a myth. However, while not all authors agree it is a myth, there is a consensus that it is difficult to achieve.

Chapter Summary

When selecting individuals to participate in a research study, it is unusual that researchers find themselves in a position where it is possible to include the whole target population. Research studies that do use this method are, by their nature, large, costly and time consuming and so are infrequently undertaken. Thus, researchers need to select a sample that will ideally be representative of the target population, if undertaking quantitative (numerically-based) research, or will offer a richness of data on the phenomenon being explored, if engaging in qualitative (narratively-based) research. Sometimes, however, due to factors such as time constraints or access to populations, the ideal is not achievable. In these situations researchers have to use alternative methods of sample selection.

When adopting a method of sampling it is important that the rationale for choosing this approach is explained and the strengths and limitations of the method is discussed. Researchers need to demonstrate that they recognise the strengths and limitations of their sampling procedures and the implications these have for their research.

🔑 Key Points 🔑

- A sample from the population is used in research as it is more cost effective, less onerous and less time consuming than including the whole target population.
- A probability sample is used if the researcher is seeking a sample that is likely to be representative of the target population.
- Non-probability samples are less likely to be representative of the target population and are used in research when certain events arise, such as not having access to a sample frame of the population.
- Quantitative (numerically-based) research uses larger sample sizes to reduce sampling bias and the risk of Type II sampling errors.
- Qualitative (narratively-based) research studies use smaller samples as they are not seeking representative samples, but attempting to gain a greater insight into the phenomenon being explored.

7

Ethical and Legal Issues in Research

Introduction

One of the greatest challenges often faced by healthcare researchers is obtaining ethical approval to proceed with a study. This is because ethics in healthcare research is a complex subject. History has revealed, as we will discuss in this chapter, some serious breaches in ethics in past studies. These have led to the development of guidance and laws, which direct and insist on appropriate ethical and legal practices in current healthcare research. Ethical guidance, although challenging at times in its remit, is and should be, very much welcomed by the healthcare research community. This is because, not only does it provide for the safety, welfare and rights of people participating in research studies, it also offers protection to anyone planning to undertake a study. In the main, ethics in healthcare research focuses on achieving three primary objectives. These are the protection of research participants, the conduct of research that is of benefit to individuals, groups and/or society and the conduct of research that, as integral, minimises risks to research participants, ensures informed consent and maintains participant confidentiality.

The focus of this chapter is to provide you with an understanding of ethics in healthcare research. The concept of ethics and the theories underpinning it will be explored. By considering some past studies that are questionably unethical, the importance of ethics in healthcare research will be highlighted. An overview of key documents and reports that offer ethical and legal guidance on the conduct of research involving humans will be provided. Key ethical principles and their application to healthcare research will be explored. The importance, role and membership of research ethics committees will be addressed. Finally, ethical and legal issues relevant to particular research designs will be discussed.

☑ Learning Outcomes ☑

By the end of this chapter you should be able to:

- Understand the concept of ethics and briefly describe the major ethical theories
- Understand why ethics in healthcare research is important
- List key documents and reports that guide the ethical and legal conduct of health-care research
- Describe key ethical principles
- Describe the role and membership of research ethics committees
- Understand and describe ethical and legal issues specific to particular types of studies.

What is Ethics?

Defining and understanding ethics is by no means easy. It is a complex subject with associated issues often giving rise to controversy, dilemma and debate. In many ways ethics is akin to the contents of 'Pandora's box', that is, on the surface issues may appear straightforward or innocuous, but when further explored, they can have far-reaching and considerable consequences. Take for example the concept of informed consent which, as you will likely know, is a core element of all research involving humans. However, what happens when a person is unable to give consent? For example, say you wish to recruit adults, over the age of eighteen, to a study that plans to evaluate the use of massage for chronic back pain. The research setting is an urban healthcare centre and the nurses and doctors at the centre act as gatekeepers (gate-keepers in research will be discussed later in this chapter). Your study information leaflet is in English. However, as the study progresses you become aware that a number of potential participants are not receiving the study information because English is not their first language. In this sense, potential participants are being denied the opportunity to participate in your study simply because they cannot understand written English. The question you must ask now is whether this is fair or right?

Ethics is a form of moral philosophy which considers, as paramount, standards of right or good in conduct and character and in choices and decisions that you, others or groups make. Beginning in childhood where you start to learn and think about what is right or wrong or acceptable or unacceptable, ethics soon becomes a familiar part of daily life. It may concern only your personal conscience where you consider whether your own conduct, actions and the decisions you make are good or bad or right or wrong. Alternatively ethics may concern society, culture, the law and religion with the expectation that individuals conform to the standards of right or good as decided upon by others. For example, euthanasia or the assisted killing of a person who has no hope of recovery from an illness or disease, at the explicit request of the person who wishes to die, often gives rise to ethical debate. The ethics here surrounds a person's right to choose when they die and whether this is acceptable or not. In many countries, legislation has decided on this with euthanasia illegal in some and legal in others. In this sense, irrespective of your own personal views on the topic you must adhere to the standard of right or good as deemed so by the legislators in the country in which you live. It is often in scenarios such as this that differing personal or group conscience can cause proponents and opponents on an issue to collide with passionate ethical debates ensuing.

As an activity to assist you to understand the complexity of ethics, think of a healthcare issue that may have given rise recently to controversy and debate in the news or national press. Jot down the arguments describing what was right or wrong or good or bad about the issue. What were your own thoughts on the matter? What did others think? Describe what you think are the main ethical issues and the impact these may have on healthcare provision.

ACTIVITY 7.1

To assist a more comprehensive understanding of ethics in healthcare research it is necessary to consider some relevant ethical theories. It is important for you to have some awareness of these theories as they can be applied to different situations in research to inform thinking and to support decision making. The three main ethical theories discussed here are deontology, utilitarianism and virtue ethics.

Deontology

Deontology in research is concerned with duty and obligation and how these can best be met (Noble, 2007). The focus here is on the actions taken by a researcher rather than on the outcome of those actions, irrespective of what these outcomes might be. In this sense, using deontological theory to guide a study, a researcher is not simply concerned with the results of their study, rather what is right to do or what ought to be done as they set out to achieve those results. An example of using deontology to guide research might be explained by considering the issue of confidentiality. A researcher has an ethical obligation to respect participant confidentiality and privacy. Consider, however, that during the course of a study a research participant discloses information that has the potential to negatively affect their welfare and possibly bias the results of the study. The participant, however, does not want this information revealed or recorded as part of the study. An ethical dilemma now emerges. On the one hand, there is an ethical obligation to respect the wishes of the participant. On the other hand, there is an ethical obligation to uphold the participants' safety and welfare and the scientific integrity of the study. Guided by deontological theory, disclosure of the information will be favoured here as a researcher will feel he/she has a sense of duty to respond to any possible harms caused by participating in the study. This is not an easy situation. A researcher must ensure that a participant is fully aware as to why disclosure is deemed important and necessary. Having an honest and open conversation with the research participant, while simultaneously ensuring their privacy as best as is possible, might offer a safe and ethically correct solution to this dilemma.

Utilitarianism

Utilitarianism contrasts to deontology as the focus here is on the value of the consequences of what a researcher does rather on what is done or ought to be done (Ohio

Nurses Association, 2013). Using this theory there is due consideration given to the end results of research with the greatest benefit to the greatest number of people, the supporting force behind actions and decisions. The oft-quoted argument that the end justifies the means (Noble, 2007) might be used to summarise utilitarianism.

Utilitarianism is often used to guide healthcare research studies where, knowingly, a researcher might be aware that there is a potential for risk or discomfort to participants in a study but is hopeful that these are minimal in contrast to the overall benefit that may be gained from the study. An example here might be a study evaluating the use of laser therapy for a skin condition such as *acne rosacea*. A researcher might be aware that the laser therapy is likely to cause transitory pain to some participants. If successful in treating the acne, however, the risk of pain during the study might seem less important when considered in the context of the overall potential benefits, such as improved physical appearance, improved quality of life and/or psychological wellbeing. In this sense, using utilitarianism to guide research, a researcher will view a study as ethically sound where it has the potential to offer significant benefit over risk to a considerable number of people.

Virtue Ethics

Virtues are qualities or characteristics that are desirable in a person and that enable a person to behave well (Gardiner, 2003). They are concerned not only with how a person acts but also with their character. Virtues include qualities such as integrity, compassion, trustworthiness and courage. In research, virtue ethics is concerned with how a researcher, as a moral human being, behaves and the qualities of his or her character that influence decisions and judgements during a study. Gardiner (2003) argues, in using virtue ethics to guide research, a researcher will evaluate a situation, judge what is right to do and act accordingly because there is a desire to act or behave well. An example of virtue ethics in research is honesty in reporting the results of a study even when the results are not what were expected or hoped for. This may appear obvious but there are past examples of both fraudulent reporting of research and non-reporting of research that showed negative results. One well-documented example is that of Hwang Woo-suk, a professor of biotechnology at Seoul National University (Columbia University, 2011). Hwang Woo-suk was considered one of the pioneering experts in the field of stem cell research and went on to publish two papers in which he reported to have succeeded in creating human embryonic stem cells by cloning. Both papers were later editorially retracted after they were found to contain a large amount of fabricated data and fraudulent reporting. This type of behaviour in research violates the very essence of virtue ethics as it demonstrates a lack of virtue in both action and in character.

Why is Ethics Important in Research?

Between November 1945 and October 1946 a series of military trials, involving leading members of Hitler's Nazi regime, took place in Nuremberg, Germany (Overy, 2011). Included in the proceedings were charges of crimes against humanity arising from medical experiments performed on individuals held in concentration camps during World War II. These experiments were performed without the person's consent and were likely to have caused horrific pain. Worse still, many individuals subjected to these experiments either died or were permanently disabled as a direct result. The Nuremberg trials mark a significant chapter in the history of research as they resulted in the first international document that stipulated voluntary participation and informed consent as essential in all research involving humans. This document, called the Nuremberg Code, contains 10 guidance points on the ethical conduct of research in humans (visit http://history.nih.gov/research/downloads/nuremberg.pdf to view full details of the Nuremberg Code).

Since the publication of the Nuremberg Code numerous other documents have been, and continue to be, developed and revised to guide the ethical and legal conduct of research involving humans. Before we consider some of these documents you should know that the Nazi experiments were not the only experiments that involved gross misconduct under the auspice of research. History unfortunately provides us with a number of examples of ethically dubious research. To understand why ethics in research is so important it is worth considering some of these studies and the ethical issues associated with them.

The Tuskegee Syphilis Study

The Tuskegee Syphilis Study (Tuskegee University, 2013), second to the Nazi Medical Experiments, is perhaps one of the most well-known studies that breached the fundamentals of ethically correct healthcare research. The study began in 1932 and continued for forty years. The research, conducted by the U.S. Public Health Service, was intent on studying the progression of untreated syphilis in the hope of learning more about the disease. Black men in a region of Macon County were recruited to the study by being told that they would receive free tests and medical treatment for a condition known as 'bad blood', a term referred to by locals for a number of ailments including fatigue, anaemia and syphilis. The true nature of the study was never explained to the participants and, even after 1943 when penicillin was discovered as a safe and effective treatment for syphilis, study participants known to have syphilis were denied this treatment. Over the lifetime of the study, over six hundred African American men were recruited to the study. When knowledge of The Tuskegee Syphilis Study became widespread it evoked a public outcry and the study was immediately stopped. In May 1997, the then president of the United States, Bill Clinton, issued an apology to the men used in the research and to their families, admitting publicly that the U.S. government did something that was profoundly and morally wrong (Centre for Disease Control & Prevention, 2011).

The Tuskegee Syphilis Study and its outcome led to a number of changes in research practices in the US. In 1974, the National Research Act was signed into law. This ensured that researchers were now legally required to get voluntary informed consent from all individuals participating in research conducted or funded by the Department of Health, Education and Welfare. Furthermore, studies supported by the Department now had to be reviewed by an institutional review board. Since this time, U.S. ethical standards and guidelines have been reviewed and revised with assurances that efforts to ensure the highest ethical standards in research are ongoing to this day (Centre for Disease Control & Prevention, 2011).

Studies Involving Prisoners and Vulnerable Others

A number of examples of research involving vulnerable people have been documented over time. Prisoners, for example, are considered vulnerable people due to concerns over possible coercion to participate in research (McDermot, 2013). This concern is not unfounded as previous studies provide evidence of coercion. One such example involved the recruitment of eleven prisoners in Rankin State Prison in Mississippi who were subjected to dietary modifications in an effort to induce pellagra, a disease caused by a chronic lack of vitamin B3 in the diet. In exchange for taking part in the research the prisoners were promised a full pardon (Office of NIH History, 1996). Another example is a study on malaria conducted at Stateville Penitentiary in Illinois (Comfort, 2009). Subsequent reviews of this study found that prisoners taking part in the study were released, on average, two years earlier than those who did not participate.

In addition to prisoners, pregnant women, children, human fetuses and neonates are also classified as vulnerable populations (McDermot, 2013). Examples of ethical misconduct have also been found in research involving these groups. For example, in the autumn of 1999, knowledge of practices of organ and tissue retention, without parental knowledge or consent, from children who had undergone heart surgery and from babies who had died in a number of hospitals in the UK, began to emerge in the national press (BBC News, 2001; Sheach Leith, 2007). Worryingly it appeared that these practices had been going on for some time. Teaching, audit and research were provided as reasons for retaining the organs and tissue samples (Sheach Leith, 2007). Following a full enquiry, informed consent was placed firmly at the centre of subsequent recommendations and this was also given priority in an ensuing revision of the Human Tissue Act (Crown, 2004).

As a final example of unethical conduct in research involving vulnerable people, it is worth mentioning the Willowbrook hepatitis study. In this study, which was carried out in the 1950s, children at the Willowbrook School for Children with Mental Retardation were injected with a mild form of hepatitis. The theory under study was that by inducing a mild form of the disease, longer-lasting immunity from future infection might be conferred (Robinson & Unruh, 2008). Although parents gave consent for their children to participate in the study, concerns were raised over how this consent was obtained. In the first instance, a place at the Willowbrook School was highly coveted. Although denied by the researchers, there have been suggestions that the only way a child could gain a place in the school was if their parent agreed for them to become a participant in the research study (Rothman, 1982). Major ethical concerns over the use of children, in particular children with intellectual disabilities, and the associated potential risk to the child as a result of participating in the study, were raised (Beauchamp & Childress, 2013).

7.1   Thoughts and Tips

As a thought, it might be an idea to suggest to your college lecturer or teacher to dedicate a session, as part of your research module, to discuss the above research studies or any other controversial studies that you might be familiar with. This would allow you and your colleagues to have an open discussion and debate on the principle ethical issues inherent in these studies. It would also provide an interesting learning exercise for assisting you to understand ethics in research.

The above studies provide some examples of ethically controversial research. They evoke concern over issues such as informed consent, denial of treatment, misplaced risk/benefit ratios and coercion and begin to explain why ethics in healthcare research is so important. They demonstrate for us how an absence of strict ethical principles and codes of ethical conduct can compromise the safety and welfare of people participating in research. They demonstrate how people might be unfairly influenced to take part in a study because of their situation. They also demonstrate the serious risk that can be placed on participants when ethically correct practices are not adhered to. In essence, questionable ethical research can compromise a person's basic human rights.

Recommendations, guidelines and laws, arising from, and in some instances as a direct result of unethical practices, give further credence to the importance of promoting and ensuring the ethically correct conduct of research in healthcare. Current ethical guidance is varied and widespread with numerous documents publicly available. In some instances, these documents have broad international applications, such as the Declaration of Helsinki, for example. In other instances they have national or local applications, such as national Data Protection Acts.

Listed below in the box are some of the main documents that govern the ethical and legal conduct of research in healthcare. This list is not exhaustive, rather, it is provided to highlight some of the key documents that you may come across as you read research reports.

Ethical Guidance Documents

- The Declaration of Helsinki (1964)

  - This document, published by the World Medical Association, is an international document providing key ethical guidance when conducting research involving humans.

- The Belmont Report (1979)

  - In the wake of public outcry over the Tuskegee Syphilis Study, the National Research Act was signed into law in the US and the National Commission for

(Continued)

(Continued)

the Protection of Human Subjects of Biomedical and Behavioural Research was created. The Commission was given a remit to identify the basic ethical principles that should underpin the conduct of biomedical and behavioural research involving humans. The Belmont Report provides a summary of these principles as identified by the Commission.

- EU Data Protection Directive 95/46/EC (1995)

  o This European Parliament Directive provides for guidance on the protection of individuals with regards to the processing of personal data, including data on research participants. In bringing national law into line with this Directive, many EU countries have passed their own data protection laws. Examples of these include the Irish Data Protection (Amendment) Act 2003, the UK Data Protection Act 1998, the Swedish Personal Data Act 1998 and the German Federal Data Protection Act 2009.

- Council for the International Organisations of Medical Science (2002)

  o This document provides international guidance for biomedical research in humans. It provides a statement of general ethical principles and twenty-one separate guidelines. The document is largely designed for application and use in low-resource countries.

- EU Clinical Trials Directive 2001/20/EC

  o This European Parliament Directive details specific provisions regarding the conduct of clinical trials involving medicinal products in humans and includes direction on good clinical practice.

Key Ethical Principles

In reading research, an understanding of the practical application of ethics is essential. For this, you must first understand four key ethical principles that underpin healthcare research. These principles are: autonomy, beneficence, non-maleficence and justice (Beauchamp & Childress, 2013).

Autonomy

Autonomy in research refers to a person's right to choose whether or not they participate in a research study and it demands that a researcher respects that person's choice. To respect a person as an autonomous individual, Beauchamp and Childress (2013) assert that a person's right to their own views and actions, based on their personal values and beliefs must be acknowledged. In this sense, any decision made by an individual to participate in a study must be of their own making, free from coercion or other influences. Informed consent is central to the principle of autonomy in research. This means that a research participant, in giving consent, has been provided with all of the necessary information to make an informed decision, that they fully understand this information, that they are not coerced to take part in the study and that they are competent to give consent.

Study Information

As part of informed consent, the information provided to potential research participants should include:

- The name of the lead researcher and/or the research team.
- The aim of the study.
- The methods or processes involved in the study, including details of what will be expected of individuals should they decide to participate and the types of data that will be collected on them.
- Full disclosure of any potential risks, benefits or discomfort that might arise as a result of taking part in the study.
- Assurances to participants that they have a right to withdraw from the study at any time if they so wish and that, if they decide to withdraw, their subsequent care will not be affected in any way.
- Assurances to participants that all information collected on them during the study will be kept private. This should include details as to how data collected during the study will be stored safely and in confidence.
- Full disclosure of plans to publish and disseminate the research results including how participant confidentiality will be maintained when doing so.

Only when a person has had time to consider the study information, has had time to ask questions and has had all their questions answered should consent to join the study be sought. Although different recommendations might exist for the time-interval between giving information and seeking consent, this is likely to be influenced by the type of research study and can, at times, pose a significant ethical challenge. For example, recruiting people to a study on diabetes who attend a diabetic clinic every week would likely allow for a 7-day time-interval for potential participants to consider the study information. Alternatively, recruiting a person who is attending an accident and emergency department to a study evaluating two different ways of treating a dislocated shoulder would demand a much shorter time-interval between giving information and seeking consent. This would pose a challenge to recruitment as, in addition to a short time-interval between information and consent, the person is also likely to be in pain. Irrespective of the scenario, however, the ethical obligation here is to ensure that a person fully understands what they are being asked to consent to. If there is any doubt about this it would be unethical to recruit this person to the study.

Coercion

Coercion in research refers to forcing or placing undue pressure or influence on people to take part in a research study. The Nazi Medical Experiments provide one example of coercion where people were forced to take part in research. Coercion constitutes a serious breach in ethics in research as it erodes personal autonomy by diminishing or removing a person's right to fully self-determine their participation in a study.

Ensuring people are not coerced to take part in a study demands that they are willing to participate in research and do so voluntarily. One recommended and often insisted upon way of ensuring this is the use of gatekeepers in accessing potential research participants. Holloway and Wheeler (2010) describe the process of gatekeeping as one which allows or denies people access to someone or something. Gatekeepers in research can exist at organisational, professional or individual levels (Benton & Cormack, 2000). For example, if a researcher wishes to conduct a study in a particular healthcare setting, the first step in accessing that setting is to gain permission from the manager or director of that setting. This will involve making contact with the relevant professional to discuss the study and to seek permission to conduct it within their organisation. This is an essential and important first step in research as it provides for the initial contact where relationships and trust between researcher and research setting begin to be formed. The second type of gatekeeper likely to be encountered is the relevant research ethics committee (REC). This is a necessary component of research as without REC approval a study cannot proceed. A final type of gatekeeper encountered in research is a person or venue that will facilitate the distribution of the study information or who may recruit participants to the study. As researchers are likely to have a subjective and personal interest in maximising participant recruitment, and this, consciously or subconsciously, could lead to coercion, many RECs or healthcare organisations will insist that a gatekeeper is used to provide potential participants with study information and/or to recruit study participants. Individual gatekeepers may include nurses, midwives, doctors or other allied healthcare professionals working in the research setting. They may alternatively include the use of the internet or specific websites for distributing study information or they may include letters of request or poster advertisements. When using individual gatekeepers it would be normal for a researcher to include his/her contact details in the information leaflet provided and to include an open request for interested people to either contact him/her with expressions of interest to participate in the study.

Competence

Competence in research is concerned with a person's ability to give consent. To be deemed competent a person must have the ability or necessary skills to fully understand a study including any associated risks/benefits and any obligations that may arise from participating in the research. A conflict related to competence in research arises when a person is not competent to provide informed consent yet that person would be important to the research or it would be unfair not to offer that person the opportunity to participate in the study. One example of this is research involving neonates, infants and young children. In such research, potential participants are not in a position or are highly unlikely (in the case of young children) to understand what is being asked of them and their perception of risk/benefit is likely to be misplaced. Other examples include research that requires participants who are unconscious, participants who are taking certain drugs or medication that may affect their mental capacity and research where potential participants are suffering from intellectual or mental health disorders. In some cases, such as with neonates or children, it may be ethically acceptable for a parent or a legal guardian to provide consent but this may not be appropriate or feasible in all cases. In essence, each of these scenarios presents a unique ethical challenge and, in planning a study where competence to give consent might be an issue, it would be advisable for the researcher, the healthcare organisation, and/or the relevant healthcare professionals to collectively discuss how this might best be approached, with ethical guidance and/or legal documents consulted as necessary.

Beneficence and Non-maleficence

Although beneficence and non-maleficence are described as two separate ethical principles they are closely linked and are considered together here. Beneficence in healthcare research refers to acting in the best interest of research participants at all times. Simply described, it means doing or promoting 'good' in research. In contrast, non-maleficence refers to 'avoiding harm'. One of the ethical challenges in 'doing good' and 'avoiding harm' is when a conflict arises between individual risk (harm) and group or widespread gain (benefit). For example, in a study designed to determine first time mothers' views of their birth experience, there is the potential for a woman to become upset as she relays her experience and especially so if the birth was particularly traumatic for her. However, this woman's experience is important for the research as it may highlight areas of care that need to be improved. In this sense, although at a personal level the research may pose a risk to an individual participant, overall, it might identify areas for practice change that could improve the care of hundreds of women using the maternity service in the future.

Another example of challenging risk/benefit ratios in research might be adverse side effects of treatment versus overall healthcare improvement. For example, consider a scenario whereby early phase trials have shown promising results that a new chemotherapeutic cancer drug might be very effective in treating a particular type of cancer but further, larger studies involving humans are needed. The researchers are aware, however, that adverse side effects associated with treatment could be a possibility. Similarly, the researchers are aware that if the treatment is effective it has the potential to provide a cure for this type of cancer. The difficulty here is that the researchers cannot know for sure before the study begins if participants will suffer ill-effects as a result of the treatment or how bad these might be. By the same token, the researchers cannot know for sure whether the majority or all of the participants will demonstrate significant improvement or experience benefit as a result of the treatment. In this sense, planning research often requires a balancing act where potential risks and potential benefits are fully considered and weighed against each other. Healthcare researchers have an ethical obligation to ensure beneficence and non-maleficence as best as they possibly can. If the potential for risk is greater overall than the potential for benefit it would simply be unethical to proceed with the study.

Justice

Justice in research refers to equity and fairness in both research participation and in treatment of participants during the course of a study. What this means is that people from all cultures, societies, religions and ethnic groups should be treated equally during the planning and conduct of research studies. In upholding the principle of justice, decision-making around study participants should not be based on socio-economic status, accessibility or on race or creed but should be guided by considering the participants most appropriate to answer the research question. It also means that the same group of people should not be repeatedly approached to participate in research nor should the same group be targeted for multiple studies that are ongoing simultaneously. Once participants have been recruited to a study they must then be treated equally, fairly, respectfully and with due regard for their health and wellbeing. All researchers have an ethical obligation to ensure that this occurs.

Research Ethics Committee (REC)

Largely arising from unethical conduct in previous studies and developments in ethical guidance, the introduction and use of RECs became an obligatory part of the research process in the 1960s (Health Service Executive, 2008). RECs are now widely established in all countries and may exist at a national level, such as a REC within a Department of Health or at a more local level, for example, within healthcare centres such as hospitals or academic institutions such as universities. Although the remit and scope of RECs vary widely (Tully, 2000; Pinkerton, 2002; Hearnshaw, 2004), in the main, they are responsible for reviewing all research studies that involve humans. It is the responsibility of all researchers to submit their proposed study to an appropriate REC for review. This may involve submitting the proposal to a number of RECs, for example a university and a hospital(s') REC.

Role of a REC

The principle role of all RECs is to review applications for proposed research studies. RECs have responsibility for approving or rejecting studies or they might make recommendations for amendments to the study, which researchers are obliged to consider. A researcher might decide to accept these recommendations and amend the proposed study accordingly or he/she might decide to reject the recommendations. If a researcher decides on the latter he/she must provide a good reason for this and must satisfy the REC that by rejecting their recommendations the ethics of the proposed study is not compromised in any way. Once a REC is satisfied that a study poses no ethical risk, it will approve the study and issue a formal letter stating this. It is only when a researcher receives this letter that the study may proceed. Some RECs, in addition to reviewing study proposals, will have responsibilities and functions that extend beyond this. These might include monitoring the study once it has begun, offering advice and guidance on unexpected ethical issues that arise as the study progresses, follow-up once the study is completed and setting guidance or policies with regards to the ethical conduct of research in their institution or locality (World Health Organization, 2011).

Ethics in publishing demands that papers reporting on research involving humans include a description of ethical approval procedures. This should include the name of the REC, the date approval was received, approval time-frame and how consent was obtained (Bath & Watson, 2009). As an exercise, when reading research reports that involve humans, highlight the section of text that describes the ethical approval for the study. Consider how the author(s) reports this. Become aware of differences in how this is reported. As you become aware of these differences start to question whether sufficient details have been provided by the authors in their paper. If not, think about further details that you would like to see reported to satisfy you that the research has been granted appropriate ethical approval. This exercise, in addition to considering ethical issues will also assist your critique of research reports.

ACTIVITY 7.2

REC Members

Membership of RECs should consist of a number of individuals with differing knowledge, expertise and views (World Health Organization, 2009, 2011). This should include individuals with backgrounds in science and medicine which would be necessary for understanding the medical/scientific aspects of the research in addition to non-scientific members who can provide value perspectives. This might include members from the lay-community, healthcare users and/or members from the legal profession. The box below provides exemplars of members of RECs in Ireland and the UK.

Exemplars of REC Membership

REC Membership: Royal College of Physicians in Ireland (www.rcpi.ie)

- A member with training in ethics such as an ethicist, philosopher or theologian, for example.
- A member with a qualification in law.
- A member with training in statistics.
- Lay members (one or two).
- A member with experience and knowledge in healthcare such as a nurse, doctor or psychologist, for example, as appropriate.

REC Membership: The National Research Ethics Service UK (http://nres.nhs.uk)

- 7–18 volunteer members.
- At least one-third must be lay members whose main personal or professional interest is not in a research area.
- The remainder of the committee are expert or specialist members and might include hospital doctors, statisticians, pharmacists, academics, people with legal, philosophical or theological backgrounds, nurses and General Practitioners.

Ethical and Legal Issues Specific to Research Designs

Some research designs give rise to specific types of ethical and legal issues that are unique or more particular to that type of design than to other designs. While we consider some of these here it is important to know that this list is not exhaustive and you might need to consider additional issues that could be of relevance to the type of study you are reading about or planning to undertake.

Clinical Equipoise

Clinical equipoise is an ethical issue specific to randomised controlled trials. It refers to a state of uncertainty which must exist among clinicians regarding the benefits of the treatments that are being compared in a trial (Daya, 2004; Miller & Brody, 2007). It provides the moral and practical justification for conducting the trial (Weijer et al., 2000) as, without clinical equipoise, the ethical argument against randomising participants to different treatments is the potential for denying half the study participants from receiving a more effective treatment. In such circumstances, a clinician or researcher knowingly recruiting a participant to a treatment, believed by them to be inferior, is in danger of compromising the welfare of that participant. Therefore, clinical equipoise, or uncertainty, is essential before enrolling a participant into a randomised controlled trial.

Clinical Trial Registration

Clinical trial registration is specific to research that involves a randomised controlled trial or quasi-randomised trial design. In 2004, The Society for Clinical Trials announced its support for legislation that would mandate registration of all clinical trials prior to enrolment of the first participant (Dickerson et al., 2004; Ghersi & Pang, 2009). In that same year, the International Committee of Medical Journal Editors (ICMJE) issued a statement requiring registration of a clinical trial in a public trials registry at or before recruitment of the first participant as a condition of consideration for publication in all eleven ICMJE member journals (De Angelis et al., 2004). This call for trial registration stemmed from evidence of selective reporting of trials and the subsequent potential to distort the body of evidence available for clinical decision making (De Angelis et al., 2004). In May 2003, the UK Clinical Controlled Trials Group formally launched a database (www.controlled-trials.com) that met the requirements of the ICMJE. A useful feature of this database is the International Standardised Randomised Controlled Trial Number (ISRCTN) whereby each registered trial is assigned a unique number to assist in tracking all publications and reports resulting from the trial.

Sensitive Data

Researchers must acknowledge that some types of information are more sensitive than other types. Sensitive data might include a person's racial or ethnic origin, religious beliefs, physical or mental health status, sexual life and criminal conduct (The Liberty Guide to Human Rights, 2009). Collecting sensitive data is an ethical issue that can arise in a number of healthcare research designs but is more common in epidemiological studies where information from private documents such as medical records is linked with other personal demographic data such as employment, socio-economic status or police records. Sensitive data in research needs to be handled particularly carefully. This is because any leakage of this type of information could have an adverse or 'knock-on' effect for participants. While ethics in research demands that all data is handled and stored in a secure manner, extra efforts should be made to ensure secure storage of sensitive data. This might include using locked filing cabinets or boxes within locked offices to store the data. Any data held in electronic form, for example on discs or computers, should be encrypted and password protected. Researchers who collect sensitive data are likely to have contacted their Data Protection Office to seek guidance as to any legal requirements for this.

Interviewing on Sensitive Topics

Almost all qualitative research designs involve interviewing participants to collect the relevant data. Interviews that involve sensitive topics, that is topics that people generally wish to keep private or which they might find embarrassing, threatening or emotionally difficult to discuss, can be particularly ethically challenging as there is the potential for discomfort, upset or disclosure of very personal information during the process. Some examples of sensitive topics might include sexual abuse, domestic violence, death, grief or illegal behaviour. Researchers planning to interview participants on a sensitive topic must have in place measures to ensure an appropriate response to possible participant distress or upset. Some examples include undertaking training on interviewing on sensitive topics prior to commencing the study, stopping and/or discontinuing the interview should a participant become distressed, offering/engaging in debriefing on the cause of upset/distress, having contact details for appropriate external support groups and ensuring follow-up referral pathways are in place for supportive counselling should participants require and wish to avail themselves of this.

Waiver of Consent

Before research is undertaken the consent of all potential participants must be obtained. However, there are some types of research designs where the requirement for a written signed consent form could be waived. One example here is postal surveys. In this instance consent to participate in the study may be appropriate by returning completed questionnaires, replacing the need for a written consent form from those participating in the study. For this to occur, however, the process of consent must be made explicit to potential participants by clearly stating and highlighting this in the information letter distributed to them. An example of this might be to include a statement such as 'returning the enclosed questionnaire is an explicit indication of willingness and consent to participate *in the study*' (Smith et al., 2014, p.46). This form of consent has been acknowledged and accepted by RECs (Conjoint Faculties Research Ethics Board, 2000) and has been used in previous survey designs using postal questionnaires (Fewell, 2005; Smith et al., 2011; 2014).

Chapter Summary

The focus of this chapter was to provide you with some understandings of ethical and legal issues in research. Ethics is undoubtedly complex and, although numerous documents are now available to guide the conduct of ethically correct research, determining what is ethical in research also requires some moral reasoning. By exploring a number of ethical theories it is hoped that you have gained an understanding of this, how these theories might be applied to research and how they can be used to inform decisions and judgements that must be made during a research study. In this chapter, a number of unethical studies were discussed. By exploring these it is hoped that you have attained further understandings as to the importance of ethics in protecting the welfare and rights of people who participate in research studies. The described studies also highlight how vulnerable people can be used in research under the auspice of medical advancement. As healthcare professionals, we have a responsibility to advance and improve healthcare provision. Doing this through research, however, should never be to the detriment of the health, welfare and rights of people in any society. The establishment of RECs, inclusive of lay members, has assisted largely in ensuring the ethically correct planning and conduct of research studies. Added to this is the obligation of all researchers to adhere to the four ethical principles of autonomy, beneficence, non-maleficence and justice. On reading this chapter, you should have a greater understanding of these principles and of the role of RECs in healthcare research. Finally, this chapter provides a brief insight into some ethical issues that pertain to particular types of research designs. This list is not exhaustive and it would be important for you to seek further advice if you are concerned or curious regarding any particular ethical issues that might arise as you are reading research reports.

🔑 Key Points 🔑

- Ethics in healthcare research is a complex subject often giving rise to debate.
- In conducting ethically sound research three objectives must be met. These are the protection of research participants, the conduct of research that is of benefit to all concerned and the conduct of research that minimises risks to participants, ensures informed consent and maintains confidentiality.
- Three ethical theories that can be used to inform thinking and support decision-making in healthcare research are deontology, utilitarianism and virtue ethics.
- Four ethical principles which underpin healthcare research involving humans are autonomy, beneficence, non-maleficence and justice.
- All proposed studies involving humans must be reviewed by a research ethics committee (REC).
- Researchers need to consider and address any additional ethical issues that may be of relevance or unique to their particular type of research design.

Useful Online Resources

The Declaration of Helsinki: www.wma.ie
The Belmont Report: www.hhs.gov/ohrp/humansubjects/guidance/belmont.html
Information on EU Directives: http://ec.europa.eu
The National Research Ethics Service, UK: www.nres.nhs.uk/
Office of the Data Protection Commissioner: www.dataprotection.ie

8

Rigour in Research

Introduction

The strength of research findings and the impact they might have on healthcare practice, provision and policy are dependent on how well a study is designed, conducted and reported. When reviewing and reading research studies it is important that you think about the 'quality' of these studies as an indicator of whether or not the research findings should or could be applied for use in clinical practice. The importance of this is centred on the likelihood that poorly designed studies are likely also to be of low methodological quality which could compromise the studies' findings. Study findings that are compromised will not be very beneficial to healthcare practitioners who want to use these findings to make decisions in healthcare practice. Contrastingly, when studies are deemed to be of high methodological quality, practitioners can be more reassured in using these findings knowing that they have emerged from a high quality research process. In this sense, the issue of 'quality' is central to the concept of rigour in research whereby quality in study design, conduct and reporting is more likely to produce results that are robust, accurate and believable. The focus of this chapter is to explore the concept of rigour in research, including its scope and importance. The concepts of validity, reliability and trustworthiness are explored so that you might gain an understanding as to how these are used in determining rigour in research. Finally, methods for assessing whether or not a research study is rigorous, will be described.

☑ Learning Outcomes ☑

By the end of this chapter you should be able to:

- Understand the concept of rigour in research
- Understand validity, reliability and trustworthiness in research
- Describe the strategies that a researcher might use to ensure that a study is rigorous
- Describe how rigour in research might be assessed.

The Concept of Rigour

There is much debate in the literature surrounding the concept of rigour and the terminology associated with it (Mays & Pope, 1995; Golafshani, 2003; Sandelowski, 2003; Rolfe, 2006). As a concept in its own right, rigour is concerned with extreme thoroughness and accuracy. It is embedded within the characteristics of diligence, attention to detail, exactness and meticulousness. Achieving rigour or being rigorous requires strict adherence to a set of principles, methods or processes. In research, from a positivist/post-positivist perspective (quantitative inquiry), rigour is described in terms of validity and reliability. Contrastingly, in naturalistic inquiry (qualitative research), the term trustworthiness is more commonly used to describe rigour. Arguably this is a matter of lexical semantics; that is, the analysis of the meaning of words, as, irrespective of philosophical perspective, the focus here is on research that is credible, reliable, accurate and true, and the methods used to achieve this. Nonetheless, *'language is the basis on which philosophical beliefs are articulated and communicated'* (Tobin & Begley, 2004: 389). In this sense, while differing terms are used, which can cause some confusion for students, transference of these terms across research paradigms might not be appropriate (Hamberg & Johansson, 1999). When reading research papers, you will likely see that the terms validity and reliability and trustworthiness are, in the main, reserved for addressing rigour in the differing quantitative and qualitative research designs respectively. Furthermore, differing strategies are applied within the differing designs to ensure validity and reliability and trustworthiness is achieved during the research process. For this reason, in this chapter, we will discuss validity, reliability and trustworthiness separately.

Validity

In research, the term validity is concerned with whether or not a study measures/tests what it intends to measure or test. If a study is deemed to be valid, then we are more reassured that the findings are accurate, true and sound. Alternatively, if a study is deemed not to be valid, then the meaning of the results is diminished as their accuracy may be called into question. In research, there are two main types of validity: i) external validity; and ii) internal validity.

External Validity

External validity is concerned with the degree to which the findings of a study are generalisable to other groups or populations; that is, how well do the study's results extend beyond the study sample to individuals in the wider community. In determining external validity the focus of assessment should be on whether the research methods inhibit the generalisability of the study's findings to the wider population. In making this assessment, you should consider differences between the target population and the study sample (Gerhard, 2008). For example, if I wanted to conduct a study on the use of recreational drugs at a national level (the target population) it would be inappropriate to source the study sample from a population of individuals attending a drug rehabilitation centre. This is because these individuals may not represent accurately the target population and the study findings will have little meaning for anyone other than the individuals who participated in the study.

Internal Validity

Internal validity relates to 'within' study features. Ensuring internal validity in research is heavily reliant on the use of data collection tools or study instruments that enable accurate, precise and true collection of study data. The key question here is 'how valid is this instrument for measuring the phenomenon of interest'? For example, in everyday life we use scales to measure weight and we accept that kilograms are a valid measure of that weight. However, in health and social care research we are often measuring phenomena or constructs that are by their very nature imprecise. Consider, for example, how difficult it is to define Health-Related Quality of Life (HRQoL), and by association, how difficult it is to develop items in a questionnaire that claim to measure it. Because of this it is almost impossible to say an instrument is 100 per cent valid. Nonetheless, to ensure internal validity, researchers should engage in strategies that indicate the degree to which their study instrument is measuring what it claims to measure.

Ensuring Internal Validity in Study Instruments

There are four main types of study instrument validity. These are: i) face validity; ii) content validity; iii) criterion validity; and iv) construct validity. In reading research reports, such as surveys for example, or other studies where questionnaires or scales have been used, you should be able to identify in the paper information regarding the extent and type of validity testing applied. This will allow you to make judgements as to how accurate you consider the study findings to be. Where study authors fail to provide information on the validity and reliability of their study instrument, this would be considered a limitation in the reporting of the research.

ACTIVITY 8.1

As an activity, identify two papers on a similar research topic of your choice that use a questionnaire or scale for collecting study data. Identify how the authors of the paper have reported the validity of their data collection tool. Identify any major differences or similarities between the reports. Judge whether you think the study instrument is sufficiently valid. Swap your papers with a colleague or classmate and ask them to repeat the exercise. Compare, contrast and discuss your findings to see if you reached similar or different conclusions.

Face Validity

Face validity is concerned with reading over a study instrument and judging whether the items (questions) on it appear to measure what they are supposed to measure. It is considered the weakest form of validity as the entire study instrument is judged at 'face value' rather than at individual item level. In this sense, the assessment is superficial and would not be sufficient on its own as a basis for declaring a study instrument valid or invalid. In most instances, researchers use face validity in combination with another form of validity testing. A common strategy used by researchers in determining face validity is requesting experts to view their study instrument and rate, on a scale of 1–5, whether they think the instrument overall appears to measure what it is intended to measure. An instrument receiving a rate of ≥ 4 would be deemed 'face valid'.

Content Validity

Content validity provides a more thorough method for determining validity. A common approach used by researchers is to follow a framework described by Lynn (1986). Using this framework, the study instrument is distributed to a panel of experts on the topic under inquiry. The panel are requested to rate each item in the instrument for relevance in answering the research question by rating each item on a scale of 1–4 where 1 = not at all relevant, 2 = somewhat relevant, 3 = relevant and 4 = very relevant. Items that average an overall mean expert rating score of < 3 should be removed from the questionnaire.

Below, the box provides an example of validity assessment reporting in a research paper evaluating student's attitudes towards the Objective Structured Clinical Examination (OSCE) as an assessment strategy for assessing clinical competence (Muldoon et al., 2014).

Exemplar of Validity Assessment Reporting in a Research Paper

A panel of three experts on the topic of OSCEs ... conducted face and content validity assessments. Face validity involved scoring the instrument, between 1 and 5, on its overall appearance ... for measuring attitudes. Content validity ... where each item was scored for relevance on a scale of 1–4 with 1 implying 'not at all relevant' and 4 implying 'very relevant'. The mean face validity score ... was 3.8, indicating 'satisfactory' face validity. The mean content validity assessment scores for 18 of the 20 statements ranged between 3.3 and 4 indicating that these statements were considered either 'relevant' or 'very relevant'. For the remaining 2 statements ... the mean content validity assessment scores were 2.3 and 2.7 respectively. This indicated that these statements were considered 'somewhat relevant' only. Thus, they were removed from the scale. (Muldoon et al., 2014: 470).

Criterion Validity

There are two types of criterion validity: i) concurrent validity; and ii) predictive validity. Concurrent validity is used to determine the accuracy of a data collection instrument by comparing it with another data collection instrument. For example, if you wished to measure neurological development in an infant at two years of age, and, rather than using one of the many currently available instruments, you decided to develop a new instrument, you would need firstly to ensure that your new instrument will accurately do this. One way of testing this is to assess an infant using the new and the previously validated instrument at the same time. If the two instruments provide similar results in terms of the infants' neurological developmental status then the new instrument is deemed to have concurrent validity. To use the new instrument if it was not deemed to be concurrently valid would undermine the validity of the results of the assessment. In other words, you could not be confident that the developmental status of the infant as indicated by the test result is an accurate or true reflection of the infant's actual developmental status.

Alternatively, predictive validity indicates how accurately a measurement instrument or test will predict outcomes at a future time. A common example of such a test is an aptitude test where the results of the test are used to predict how well someone might perform in the future. Aptitude tests have been used during employment selection processes, for example. Those who perform well in the test are likely to have a greater chance at being offered the job with the idea being that their job performance will be better than those who score poorly in the test. For the aptitude test to be deemed valid it must first be tested to ensure that the results from it are truly reflective of future performances. This could be done by assessing performance and mapping back to the aptitude test results to determine if they correlate accurately. This might take a number of years to achieve. If however, both results correlate sufficiently then the test may be deemed to have predictive ability and thus be used with confidence from that point forward.

Construct Validity

Constructs refer to images, ideas or theories, often complex, which do not necessarily emerge from empirical science. In healthcare, for example, HRQoL would be deemed a construct. HRQoL is almost impossible to define as it may mean very different things to different people and differ at different times in people's lives depending on their particular circumstances and their perceptions of these. Yet there are numerous questionnaires that attempt to measure HRQoL. To ensure that these questionnaires measure what they intend to measure, validity assessments may be applied as they are being developed. Construct validity attempts to ensure that there is a congruity between the variables of the conceptual framework (the idea of what HRQoL is or should be) and how the researcher plans to measure these (items in the scale that will be used to measure HRQoL). This form of validity testing is highly complex and beyond the scope of this chapter. To find out more about this type of validity we would suggest sourcing an advanced research text book that specifically focuses on validity testing in quantitative inquiry.

Reliability

Referring to someone as a reliable person brings to mind someone whom we can depend on or who is consistent. The concept of reliability in research is similar and is concerned with establishing the extent to which a study, or more specifically, an instrument used in a study, consistently measures what it intends to measure. To return to the weighing scales example, reliability is concerned with determining if the measure of weight is consistent each time it is used. Of course most of us are aware that we may get different readings of weight when two different scales are used because of how they are calibrated. This is an important point when considering two scales in health and social care research that claim to measure the same phenomenon. For example, there is continuing debate in the research literature about the use of generic HRQoL scales or disease-specific scales. They both claim to measure HRQoL but may get slightly different results because of possibly different emphasis in the items used. A number of tests may be applied to determine the reliability of an instrument. The generally accepted cut-off reliability values are:

- Weak reliability: 0.00–0.40
- Moderate reliability: 0.41–0.60
- Strong reliability: 0.61–0.80
- Very strong reliability: 0.81–1.00

8.1   Thoughts and Tips

When reading research papers, it is worth noting that reliability is often denoted in research papers by the symbol 'r' with the reliability result presented after this symbol.

Three generally accepted ways of ensuring instrument reliability are: i) stability; ii) internal consistency; and iii) equivalence. The choice of reliability testing might be dependent on the type of study instrument being used and the items in it.

Ensuring Reliability in Study Instruments

Stability

The stability of an instrument refers to the degree to which an instrument generates similar findings from the same (or similar) group of individuals on different occasions. If a study instrument can demonstrate stability this indicates that it would be reliable, for example, for use in populations in different regions in a country or in different countries, where the target population would be characteristically similar (e.g. a group of teenagers attending high school, a group of individuals suffering from dementia, or a group of patients suffering from a particular cancer) to the population upon which the instrument was initially tested. The most common way to establish instrument stability is to subject it to a test-retest exercise. The box below provides a worked example of how this can be done using the OSCE example from earlier (Muldoon et al., 2014).

Example of a Test-retest Exercise

- The study sample was a group of 3rd year midwifery students who had undertaken an OSCE assessment.
- A Likert scale was developed to measure students' attitudes where students rated their agreement with statements on the scale using values from 1 (strongly disagree) to 5 (strongly agree).
- To determine stability, the instrument was administered to another group of students who had undertaken this OSCE the previous year. The overall mean total student score, for each item on the scale, was calculated and entered into the computer package SPSS. This was considered the test phase.
- Two weeks later, the same group of students were asked to complete the instrument again (the retest phase). The mean student scores for each item on the scale were again calculated and entered into SPSS.
- Using a statistical test called Spearman's correlation co-efficient, the relationship between the test and retest scores was calculated (SPSS automatically calculates this for you). A result of 0.871 was demonstrated, indicating excellent instrument reliability.

8.2   Thoughts and Tips

Establishing instrument stability should be done when researchers are developing a new instrument for use in a study. Where researchers are replicating or conducting a study similar to one that has been completed previously on the same topic, the reliable instrument used in the earlier study could be considered for use. Permission must be granted for this by the previous study's researchers.

Internal Consistency

Internal consistency is used to determine the degree to which items on a questionnaire measure a particular variable. It is often used for study instruments where multiple item scores are added to calculate a composite (overall) score of the variable under measurement. For example, if a researcher wished to measure depression, the instrument or scale used would likely contain a number of questions that measure various aspects of depression. As you would expect that all of the items are indicators of depression, you would also expect that each item in the scale would correlate with each of the other items. If some items in the scale are worded poorly or are not indicators of depression then they might weaken the internal consistency of the scale. Using the OSCE example once again, the internal consistency of the attitude scale was calculated using Cronbach's alpha, a common measure for this type of reliability. This was done by using the test study sample's mean scores for each item in the scale (as described in the box above). The reliability analysis function in SPSS was then used for computing the alpha result. Acceptable values for Cronbach's alpha range from 0.70 to 0.95; although for purposes of research, such as the one described in the OSCE study, a Cronbach's alpha of between 0.60 and 0.70 has been reported as acceptable (Bland & Altman, 1997). Cronbach's alpha for the OSCE instrument was reported as 0.676. This would indicate moderate to strong internal consistency of the instrument for measuring student attitudes towards the OSCE.

Equivalence

Equivalence, as a form of reliability, is usually more applicable in observational studies, where more than one researcher is observing something or performing some activity to obtain data to answer the research question. Of key importance here is collection of data by each researcher in the same way. This is referred to as interrater reliability and if it is not ensured then the results become unreliable. Consider, for example, a study in which an individual's pulse rate is measured immediately before and one hour after administering a medication to determine if the medication has any effect on pulse rate. Researcher A determines the pulse rate by counting for 15 seconds and then multiplying by 4. Researcher B, on the other hand, determines the pulse rate by counting for 1 full minute. This could result in subtle differences in the data obtained by the researchers, which has the potential to reduce the reliability of the findings. Similarly, reliability can be affected if the same researcher measures the pulse rate in different ways on different study participants at different time points. This is referred to as intrarater reliability. Equivalence in research is usually determined by calculating the percentage agreement, commonly using Cohen's Kappa test (McHugh, 2012), in the measurements obtained by the different researchers in the study. In the pulse rate example, interrater reliability might be achieved by assessing the percentage agreement of a pulse measurement on one participant by two or more researchers. If the percentage equivalence is low between the raters, that is < 40 per cent or 0.40, this would indicate weak equivalence and must be addressed before collecting further data.

A final point of note is that validity and reliability are desirable in all measures but this is not always the case. Instruments can be valid in that they measure the phenomenon of interest but they may not be reliable as the results obtained may not be consistent. Think back to the weighing scales example where the scale accurately measures weight (valid) but the results are inconsistent whereby the scale registers a different result on each occasion due to some flaw in the scale. Equally, an instrument can be reliable but not valid in that it produces consistent results but does not accurately measure the phenomenon of interest, for example, the weighing scale gives a consistent weight on each occasion but this weight is inaccurate.

Trustworthiness

The word trustworthiness is usually applied to rigour in qualitative research studies. It is similar to validity and reliability in that the questions asked are the same: can we trust the findings of the study and how do we know them to be reliable and true? Due to the very contextual and subjective nature of qualitative inquiry, establishing trustworthiness can be challenging. While there are different approaches to ensuring trustworthiness in qualitative research (Creswell, 2009), the most common approach used is based on the criteria developed by Guba and Lincoln of credibility, dependability, transferability and confirmability (Guba, 1981; Lincoln & Guba, 1985).

Credibility

Credibility attempts to demonstrate that the findings from studies and their interpretations accurately describe the participants' experiences. It is likened to internal validity in quantitative research (Shenton, 2004). Varied strategies are used by researchers to ensure credibility and these should be described in research reports. Examples of these strategies are prolonged engagement, triangulation and member checking.

Prolonged engagement involves the investment of a sufficient amount of time in data collection by the researcher. This is especially important in research such as ethnography where culture is being observed. Limited time in the field will reduce the credibility of the data as one could argue whether culture can be sufficiently explored without spending a considerable amount of time in the field. Triangulation, alternatively, involves the use of multiple referents in determining findings. For example, the researcher may use observation, focus groups and individual interviews to collect data. Use of all three will assist researchers to gain a deeper and more accurate understanding of the phenomenon under investigation. Member checking, as another strategy for establishing credibility, involves a check of the data by someone other than the researcher and might likely involve the research participants. This may involve showing study participants preliminary results and obtaining their reactions to initial interpretations and findings.

Dependability

Dependability is concerned with the stability of study data over time and conditions. It is akin to the criterion of reliability in positivist inquiry (Shenton, 2004). Strategies that a researcher might employ here include the use of several researchers in dealing with the data separately. In this sense, two or more independent inquiries are performed following which the data, how it is interpreted and the conclusions drawn from it, can be compared and contrasted. This is known as stepwise replication and it would be expected that the results and conclusions drawn would be similar across the independent inquiries. Scrutiny of data and any relevant supporting documentation by an external reviewer might also help determine dependability.

Transferability

Transferability refers to the extent to which a study's findings can be transferred to other settings or groups. If as a reader of research you can demonstrate or determine that the findings of a study are applicable to other groups or in other settings, the study is said to have transferability. To achieve transferability, the research report must provide sufficient descriptive data (thick description), including precise details of what was done in the field, to allow for the reader to evaluate the applicability of the study's findings to other contexts.

Confirmability

The criterion of confirmability is concerned with the accuracy, relevance and meaning of data in interpretivist/constructivist inquiry. It is achieved by the researcher leaving a clear trail, often referred to as an 'audit trail' as to how the data and evidence were managed and how conclusions were derived (Streubert & Carpenter, 2011). Researchers often maintain a reflective journal or detailed field notes to assist with this. This allows an independent auditor to review these documents and the research findings and to come to conclusions about the data. Where independent auditor conclusions reflect those of the researcher then the findings can be considered 'confirmed'.

Assessing Rigour in a Research Study

Rigour in a study can be assessed both informally and formally, although for academic assignments, research-related reports and evaluating research for use in healthcare practice, it is recommended that the latter should more often be used. Informal assessment implies reading a study publication or a research paper while mentally asking oneself some key questions related to the quality of the study and perhaps noting down areas where rigour seems compromised. Formal assessment, alternatively, involves the use of a framework or quality assessment tool to determine the extent to which the study conforms to standards required for methodological rigour.

One such method of formally assessing the quality of research is through critical appraisal or research critique. Research critique is an assessment of a study's merits and limitations. In critiquing research an assessment of the quality of the study can be inadvertently determined. Critiquing and evaluating research studies is explored in Chapter 12.

A second method of formally assessing rigour in research is to use a specifically designed and validated formal quality assessment tool. These tools, of which there are many, are used to assess the methodological quality of a study. The quality assessment tool guides you through an assessment process which culminates in a judgement as to whether the research is of low, moderate or high quality. As different studies adopt different designs to answer specific research questions, and because the methods employed in these studies are necessarily different also, diverse quality assessment tools specific to different research designs have been developed. In choosing a quality assessment tool specific to the study design, it is important also to choose a tool that has been validated for its purpose. Similar to ensuring validity in research, using a validated quality assessment tool will increase rigour in the formal quality assessment process.

Table 8.1 provides examples of formal quality assessment tools and the type of study designs to which they are applicable. A list of other tools available for use (including reporting quality assessment tools), is available from the EQUATOR

Network (www.equator-network.org), an organisation concerned with enhancing the quality and transparency of health research.

Table 8.1   Examples of formal quality assessment tools

Assessment Tool	Application and Description
Cochrane Risk of Bias Tool (http://www.cochrane.org)	Used by the Cochrane Collaboration and others for assessing quality (bias) in experimental research. Components such as sequence generation, allocation concealment, blinding, and other sources of bias are rated on a yes, no, cannot tell/unclear scale. An overall high (yes), low (no), or unclear risk of bias judgement is made
"The Quality Assessment Tool For Quantitative Studies" developed by the Effective Public Health Practice Project (EPHPP, 2009) (http://www.ephpp.ca/Tools.html)	The EPHPP quality assessment tool assists in assessing randomised trials and non-randomised studies for potential sources of bias. Components such as bias in selection or allocation, blinding, confounding, methods used for data collection, withdrawals from the study, analysis and intervention integrity are assessed. Following assessment, a study is given an overall rating of strong quality (no weak ratings), moderate (one weak rating) or weak (two or more weak ratings)
Newcastle Ottawa Scale (Wells et al., 2014)	Applicable to non-randomised studies such as observational cohort studies. This scale contains 8 items within 3 core categories of selection, comparability and outcome. A star is awarded to items in each category and a quality judgement is made based on the total number of stars allocated in the scale
Evidence for Policy and Practice Information and Coordinating (EPPI) Centre at the Institute of Education in London (https://eppi.ioe.ac.uk)	The EPPI-Centre provides examples of various tools used in their work on systematic reviews. One such example is a 12-item rating scale that can be applied to quantitative and qualitative research designs
Critical Appraisal Skills Programme (CASP) – Quality Assessment Tools (http://www.casp-uk.net/)	CASP provide examples of checklists for a variety of study designs, both qualitative and quantitative, and for systematic reviews. By completing a study design specific checklist, an assessment of study rigour is determined
AMSTAR (Shea et al., 2007)	The AMSTAR tool was developed and validated to assess the methodological quality of systematic reviews. It contains 11 items with yes, no, cannot answer and not applicable response options

Chapter Summary

The focus of this chapter was to provide you with an understanding of rigour in research. Rigour, which can be a complex concept to understand, essentially relates to quality in research. Ensuring high quality in research design, conduct and reporting will ensure rigour in research. The terms validity, reliability and trustworthiness are central to rigorous research. While these terms are differentially used across research paradigms, their meanings are similar in that they are measures of accuracy, consistency, trust and truth. By providing you with a description of these terms and the criteria within them, this should assist you to understand these when reading research papers. It is also important to understand that authors should report in detail their efforts to achieve rigour in their research. Not to do so should result in you questioning the rigour of the research study. Where research is deemed not to be rigorous, it is important that you proceed with caution, or not at all, in using these findings for informing your healthcare practice. An overview of formal quality assessment tools was provided in this chapter. This list is not exhaustive, rather it was provided so that you might understand that there are assessment tools available for use, that they can be specific to study designs and that they can be very helpful in assessing formally the methodological rigour of a study so that judgements on the quality of a study can be made.

☜──◖ Key Points ◗──☞

- Rigour in research is closely connected with the concept of 'quality'.
- Studies that are conducted rigorously are more likely to produce results that are more accurate, credible and true.
- In quantitative and qualitative inquiry different terms are applied to describe rigour. These are validity and reliability and trustworthiness respectively.
- To ensure rigour a researcher must subject their study instrument to various tests or perform specific activities (for example, expert review for content relevance, test-retest analyses, audit trial, triangulation and member checking) to ensure methodological rigour is achieved during the research process.
- Formal quality assessment tools are available and can be used to assess whether or not a research study is rigorous.

Useful Online Resources

www.equator-network.org/
www.ephpp.ca/index.html
www.nccmt.ca/registry
www.casp-uk.net/
https://eppi.ioe.ac.uk

9

Data Collection in Research

Introduction

Choosing the most appropriate method of collecting data is fundamental to undertaking a successful study. This chapter presents an outline of the most commonly used methods of data collection in healthcare research. The methods of data collection presented include measurement scales, questionnaires, interviews, observation and documentary sources. It is important to note that a clear distinction between methods is not possible because each may use elements of others. For example, a questionnaire can be administered in an interview situation and vice versa, and observation can include the use of a questionnaire. Variations, strengths and limitations of each of the methods are described.

☑ Learning Outcomes ☑

By the end of this chapter you should be able to:

- Outline the commonly used methods of data collection
- Describe the characteristics of the various methods of data collection
- Explain the types of data that are produced from the range of data collection methods
- Align the data collection method with the aim or purpose of a research study.

What is Data Collection?

Data collection is simply the process used by researchers to collect the necessary information to answer the research question or meet the aim of the study. Ensuring that the chosen method of data collection answers the research question/aim is fundamental to the credibility of a study. Therefore, data collection is the centre-piece of a research study because without meaningful data the study itself is worthless.

While choosing the most appropriate method of data collection begins with the research question it is possible to answer similar questions with different types of data. Remember in Chapter 1 we stated that members of any scientific community tend to have collective beliefs about what constitutes knowledge and how research is and should be undertaken. These shared beliefs tend to influence the type of research questions that are posed, the research designs most commonly used and by association the type of data that will be collected. In other words, researchers in developing their research questions come with some ideas of the type of information they wish to collect. For an illustration of the most common methods of data collection see Table 9.1.

Table 9.1   Common methods of data collection

Questionnaire	• Self-administered (postal, online, telephone)
	• Face-to-face
	• Observation (check list or rating scale)
Interview	• Face-to-face
	o Structured
	o Semi-structured
	o Unstructured
	• Group (focus group)
Observation	• Participant observation
	• Non-participant observation
Documentary sources	• Documents in the public domain
	• Documents with restricted access, e.g. patients' medical records, organisation records
	• Published materials, e.g. journal articles, previous research, books

Questionnaires, Tests and Scales

Questionnaires have become a ubiquitous part of modern life and are used most commonly to survey large groups of people about their opinions. Most adults will have taken part in some poll or survey that range from the obligatory Census Polls to our views or experiences of using a particular product. Also, many of us will have completed tests and measures of personality, intelligence and/or undergone psychometric testing. While these tests and scales are technically not questionnaires, they can often be found within or referred to as questionnaires and Knight (2002: 80) states they can be treated as a 'special form of questionnaire'.

Purpose of Questionnaires

In healthcare, questionnaires, tests and scales are adopted in a wide range of studies and for a multitude of purposes. In research, they are known as 'instruments' or 'tools' and are used to measure or test an array of phenomena such as knowledge, attitudes, beliefs, intentions, cognition, functional status, emotion/ mood, health status, quality of life and behaviour (Botti & Endacott, 2008; Jones & Rattray, 2010).

As described in Chapter 5, depending on the nature and purpose of the study, questionnaires can be used to simply describe a situation as it currently exists or they can address more complex issues such as associations or comparisons as in correlational and comparative research. For example, a questionnaire could be used to test diabetic patients' knowledge of their condition (descriptive) and nothing else. However, if the researchers wanted to use this information to see if there is any relationship between individual attributes and knowledge (correlational/comparative) they may also collect some demographic data, for example, age, educational status, literacy skills and examine if any these factors have any influence.

Questionnaires, tests and scales are the primary method of data collection in experimental and quasi-experimental studies and they are used as a means to test whether or not the intervention has had an impact. These measures are largely associated with outcome and you will see them described as such in many studies. For example, in healthcare intervention studies, a commonly used measure to determine the effect of an intervention (outcome) is improved Health-Related Quality of Life (HRQoL). In order to assess HRQoL, the researchers will choose an appropriate tool, of which there are many and measure the participants' HRQoL before and after the intervention. Alternatively, they may administer the intervention to one group (experimental group) and give usual care to another group (control group) and measure HRQoL in both groups. The 'difference', if there is one, may then be attributed to the effect of the intervention.

Format of Questionnaires

Given the range of purposes for which a questionnaire can be used the format and the types of questions posed within it will vary accordingly. For the most part though, questionnaires use forms of closed questions such as two-way (yes/no), multiple choice, ranking, scaling, contingency, checklist (see Table 9.2). Sometimes, open-ended questions are included where respondents are given the opportunity to expand upon some of their answers. While this might illuminate some of the answers, it creates difficulties in terms of analysis. Questionnaires may also include what are known as vignettes, whereby a given situation is described and followed by a list of related questions. For example, vignettes can be useful in assessing practitioners' knowledge of a clinical situation.

Very commonly, questionnaires use scales of which there are many but the most common and familiar are Likert Scales, which measure level of agreement with pre-defined statements. Level of agreement is indicated on a scale from 'strongly agree' to 'strongly disagree' with five options being the most common although four, seven and nine have been used also. Another scale that is used sometimes is the Guttman Scale, whereby the respondent ticks statements with which they agree. The Guttman Scale is a cumulative one as it consists of a hierarchy of items. Therefore, when a person ticks a statement with which they agree it is likely that they will also agree with statements lower down in the hierarchy. Further details on scales can be sourced at www.socialresearchmethods.net/kb/scaling.php.

Table 9.2   Types and format of questions

Two-Way or Dichotomous	Yes/No, True/False, Male/Female
Multiple-choice	One answer to be chosen from a number of options
Contingency/Filter	Where a question is asked and depending on the response (yes or no) respondents are directed to a particular question, e.g. Do you drink alcohol? If the answer is 'NO' then the respondents skips subsequent questions about the amount of alcohol consumed
Ranking	Ranking items, e.g. in order of preference/importance
Scaling	Choosing an option from a range, which corresponds most closely with views/beliefs/feelings about the statement, e.g. indicating level of agreement from 'strongly agree' to 'strongly disagree'
Checklist	Ticking items on a pre-designed checklist, e.g. Activity List, Performance Checklist

The format or type of question used in a questionnaire is important because they indicate the 'type or level of data' that will be produced and therefore how the data should be interpreted and the type of statistical analysis that can be undertaken. There are four levels of data that are defined as nominal; ordinal; interval and ratio. (see Table 9.3 and Chapter 10).

Table 9.3   Levels of data

Nominal	• Lowest level of measurement • Assigning numbers to distinguish one category from another, e.g. gender • They do not have a numerical value so they cannot be compared or treated mathematically
Ordinal	• Where named attributes are on a scale but given a number, e.g. strongly agree = 5 and strongly disagree = 1 • Differs from nominal in that there is a sense of ordering, i.e. lower to higher. But the difference between the numbers is not equal, e.g. difference between 1 and 2 cannot be said to be the same as between 3 and 4 and so on
Interval	• In interval data, the distance between the assigned numbers is equivalent, e.g. degrees of temperature • However, there is no absolute zero, e.g. there are minus degrees of temperature • Therefore, it cannot be said that one value is worth exactly half of another value, e.g. 10°C is not exactly half as warm as 20°C
Ratio	• A ratio scale is an interval scale with an absolute zero, e.g. where a minus does not exist, e.g. height, weight, age in years, blood pressure, length

Deciding on a Questionnaire

While researchers can and do develop their own questionnaires to answer their research questions, in reality many choose one that already exists and in many cases adapt it slightly for their purposes. For example, if a researcher is interested in measuring HRQoL there are a large number of pre-existing generic and disease/condition-specific tools that can be used and will ultimately save the researcher a good deal of time. This is because developing a new instrument is a protracted and complex process that involves defining what is to be measured, developing a list of items that represent the phenomenon and undertaking tests to ensure the final instrument is valid and reliable ever before it can be used to collect data.

Regardless of whether researchers develop their own or use a pre-existing questionnaire there are two fundamental questions that should be answered. Firstly, is the questionnaire measuring what it is supposed to measure (validity) and does it produce consistent results each time it is used (reliability)? In any research study you are reading there should be an explanation of how these two concepts were established or confirmed (see Chapter 8 for further information on validity and reliability).

Administration of Questionnaires

The underpinning notion of questionnaires is the collection of standardised data from a large sample where the same questions or observations are applied in every case ensuring consistency and objectivity. They can be administered once, before and after (an intervention) or on several occasions over a specified period of time depending on the purpose of the study. They can be completed in a variety ways that include self-administered (postal, online), face-to-face and observation, the latter most often using a checklist. Completion of structured questionnaires over the telephone is commonly undertaken but because there is direct interaction between the researcher and the participant, they are considered in the section on interviewing below.

Self-administered questionnaires are those where the research participants complete the questionnaire usually without the presence of the researcher. In the past, postal questionnaires were the norm but to a certain degree this has been superseded by the online method. Both postal and online questionnaires tend to suffer from poor response rates. These can be as low as 30 per cent (Gerrish & Guillaume, 2006) and it is necessary for researchers to outline the strategies they adopted to maximise responses. In addition, when administered through the post or online, issues of non-completion of individual items cannot be addressed, particularly if the questionnaire is an anonymous one.

Structured questionnaires are sometimes administered in face-to-face interviews (see section on interviews) and benefit from a higher response rate as the researcher can clarify items and ensure the questionnaire is completed as it should be. However, they tend to be more expensive to administer.

Observation using a structured questionnaire is also used as a method of data collection. In these instances, researchers usually act in the role of 'complete observer' (see section on Observation) where the focus is on observing and recording specific behaviours, such as an activity checklist. In these situations there is little or no interaction with those being observed.

Interviews

Interviews have become an increasingly common method of data collection in health and social care research. Interviewing is used in many different types of studies where it can be the main form of data collection or can be used in conjunction with other methods. There is considerable variation in the structure and depth of interviews but their emergence as an increasingly popular method of data collection is largely associated with their widespread use in studies that gather narrative data. Interviews can offer insights into the experiences, perceptions or views of people about a particular phenomenon.

Format of Interviews

Interviews are broadly classified as structured, semi-structured or unstructured. Structured interviews, as the name implies use an interview schedule where the questions are standardised both in terms of content and the order in which they are asked with the aim of being consistent. The questions are pre-planned, that is, they are constructed before the data collection process begins. Therefore, it is likely that some knowledge about the topic already exists. In some situations a pre-existing questionnaire may be used but instead of being self-administered (completed by the participant) it is administered by the researcher who therefore controls the interaction. These types of interviews can be likened to the survey questionnaire where the questions are designed to seek responses that can be measured statistically, usually at the level of description. The only difference may be the inclusion of some open-ended questions, which can be used to supplement or illuminate the numerical data.

Structured interviews tend to be used in situations where participants cannot read or understand the written word or who otherwise may not be able to complete a questionnaire. They are used also as part of the development or testing of the feasibility of a questionnaire. For example, patients are increasingly included in each stage of the development of instruments (questionnaires) to measure disease specific Health-Related Quality of Life (HRQoL). As part of this process, they may be involved in a structured interview with the researcher where the intended or draft questionnaire is completed. Following completion, the patient may then be given the opportunity to comment on the questions or highlight important areas that may have been missed.

Semi-structured interviews are more flexible and tend to use an interview guide rather than a strict schedule. This means that although the researcher comes to the interview with pre-determined discussion topics, he/she can respond also to issues or views raised by the participant. Developing a topic guide is a highly skilled activity for a number of reasons. Primarily and as in all research studies, the researcher has an interest in the topic and is likely to have pre-conceived ideas about it. While this is to be expected, there is a risk when using semi-structured interviews that the interview guide could be based solely on these pre-conceived ideas. This may ultimately result in data that addresses only those things the researcher considers important and possibly omitting aspects that were not part of his/her experience or that he/she considers unimportant. Therefore, a fundamental aspect of any study using semi-structured interviews is a rigorous review of the literature to develop a guide that is not only informed by the researcher's experience but by previous research, standards and practice guidelines and existing theories.

Unstructured interviews are those that are the most flexible, least directional and are focussed on the participants' perspectives of a phenomenon. Studies that use unstructured interviews are exploratory and often associated with a topic about which little is known. Even though these types of interviews are termed 'unstructured' in reality the researcher usually begins by introducing the topic following which the participant is asked to talk about their experiences or views of the phenomenon being studied. Questions that begin with 'tell me about …' often form the starting point. The subsequent discussion is largely directed and controlled by the participants with the researcher's role being one of facilitator. These types of interviews are also the most detailed and in-depth and therefore they generate the richest data. Also, they often involve meeting more than once possibly over several weeks or months.

Conducting Interviews

Interviews can be conducted with individuals and in groups, the latter usually being equated with what are known as focus group interviews. For the most part individual or one-to-one interviews are conducted face-to-face or on the telephone but with technological advancements there has been a rise in the use of electronic media such as email and online chat rooms as well as online communication networks and video conferencing. In reading a study that has used interviews, you should be able to discern why the researchers chose the approach they did. For example, if a researcher wants to interview people who live in inaccessible areas then a form of online interview might have been adopted. Alternatively, if potential participants do not have internet access, face-to-face or telephone interviews might be more appropriate.

Individual Face-to-face Interviews

Individual face-to-face interviews are used in structured, semi-structured and unstructured interviews. See the two boxes below for examples of how interviews have been used in research. Generally, they require well developed interpersonal skills on the part of the researcher to establish a rapport and facilitate the participants' telling of their experiences. Nonetheless, they are advantageous in that they allow the researcher to contextualise the interview and observe as well as listen. In addition, the researcher can respond immediately to any questions and offer clarification of the purpose of the research in terms the participants understand. They are also useful for collecting data from those who have limited literacy skills.

However, individual face-to-face interviews also have disadvantages. They can be seen by participants as intrusive or can evoke strong emotions that must be handled by the researcher. They are the most demanding in terms of time and possibly travel to various locations and therefore can be expensive compared to other methods. Moreover, the more flexible and in-depth the interview, the more data is likely to be generated, which has implications for the analysis phase of the study.

Example of How In-depth Interviewing was used in a Research Study

Title: Living with chronic pancreatitis: a qualitative study (Cronin & Begley, 2013)

Aim of the study: To develop an understanding of what it means to live with chronic pancreatitis using Gadamerian philosophical hermeneutics.
Objectives:

- Illuminate the everyday contextualised and culturally situated lives of those living with chronic pancreatitis.
- Explicate the meaning of living with chronic pancreatitis as a basis for understanding and interpretation by others.

Interviews:

- A total of 41 individual or joint interviews involving:
- Multiple, unstructured, audio-taped interviews with 14 persons with chronic pancreatitis with each person's participation lasting between four and six months.
- Interviews with five close family members (two wives, one mother, one daughter, one sister), three of which were joint interviews with the primary participant.
- Diary data from one participant.

Example of How Semi-structured Interviewing was used in a Research Study

Title: Women's and care providers' perspectives of quality prenatal care: a qualitative descriptive study (Sword et al., 2012)

Purpose of the study: To explore women's and care providers' perspectives of quality prenatal care in order to inform the development of items for a new instrument, the Quality of Prenatal Care Questionnaire.

Interviews:

- A total of 80 interviews (40 pregnant women and 40 care providers) from five sites.
- Semi-structured interview schedule based on Donabedian's systems-based model of quality healthcare (Structure, Process, Outcome)
- Opening Question: 'What does quality pre-natal care mean to you?'
- Subsequent questions based on Structure, Process, Outcome

  o Structure questions related to the physical setting and staff characteristics
  o Process questions related to clinical care (application of medical and other sciences and technology to deliver the best healthcare) and interpersonal processes (social and psychological interactions between healthcare professionals and those using the service)
  o Outcome questions related to user satisfaction with the service.

Group Face-to-face Interviews (Focus Groups)

Group, face-to-face interviews (focus groups) are a useful means of gaining insight into the collective views of a group of people who share a common characteristic or experience that is the focus of the research (Ellis, 2010). The researcher may access a pre-existing group or may establish one for the specific purpose of the research. Although there is no definitive agreement on the ideal number in a focus group they usually involve between four and twelve people. Holloway and Wheeler (2010) suggest that six is probably an optimal number as it is large enough to obtain a number of perspectives but not too large as to become unmanageable.

Focus group interviews are characterised by a social and dynamic interaction. Members of the group engage in discussion that stimulates and builds upon what has gone before. In this way, new ideas can emerge and there is potential for members of the group to alter or change their views about the topic, while in the midst of the discussion. Focus groups are also an efficient means of collecting data from a number of people, are suitable for those who do not wish to be interviewed individually and those that have limited literacy skills.

In a focus group, the researcher usually adopts a role referred to as facilitator or moderator. This necessitates highly developed skills in facilitating group discussion. In this role, the researcher establishes ground rules with the group, introduces the topic for discussion, asks questions, manages the discussion and tries to ensure all members of the group contribute. Many focus groups have a second person who adopts the role of observer, taking account of aspects such as body language, behaviour within the group and responses to questions.

One of the major disadvantages of focus groups is ensuring every member contributes to the discussion. There can be a tendency for one or more persons to dominate the discussion and if not managed by the facilitator can result in members of the group submitting to the views of the more dominant members.

A practical problem encountered in focus groups is one related to recording the group discussion. If more than one person speaks at the same time, no matter how good the equipment, it will be difficult to decipher what an individual has said. So, in addition to managing the overall discussion, the facilitator has to ensure, where possible, that only one person is speaking at any given time. See the box below for an example of a study that used focus groups as a means of collecting data.

Example of How Focus Group Interviewing was used in a Research Study

Title: The experience of fatigue in people with inflammatory bowel disease: an exploratory study (Czuber-Dochan et al., 2013)

Aim of the study: to explore inflammatory bowel disease fatigue, its impact on daily life and the strategies used to ameliorate the symptom, as described by those who experience it.

Interviews:

- Five focus groups involving 46 participants 15 of whom were men (4–12 in each group) with each lasting 90–120 minutes and digitally recorded and transcribed verbatim.

- Trigger questions devised and based on existing evidence, for example:.

  o What fatigue feels like
  o What it means to the person
  o Different types of fatigue
  o Triggers of fatigue
  o Managing the fatigue
  o Discussing fatigue with others
  o The impact of fatigue on life
  o The effect of other factors on fatigue, for example, pain.

Telephone Interviewing

Telephone interviewing is used most commonly with structured interviews and is seen as a useful means of conducting survey work. They have a higher response rate than postal questionnaires and are cheaper to conduct than face-to-face interviews. Telephone interviews also provide the researcher with the opportunity to clarify the questions and ensure that all the questions are answered, which is not possible when using a self-complete or self-administered questionnaire. Where a topic is potentially sensitive, they can be perceived as less threatening and participants are likely to find it easier to refuse to answer questions. However, the gains in terms of response rate and cost must be calculated against the loss of the interpersonal interaction in face-to-face interviews.

Electronic Interviewing

In recent years, there has been an increase in the use of online technology to gather data from individuals and groups. These can be broadly divided into 'synchronous' and 'asynchronous' types. The primary difference between the two is whether or not they occur in real-time. Synchronous online interviewing occurs in 'real-time' and the settings for discussion are usually chat rooms, discussion boards or online virtual focus groups. Asynchronous interviewing does not occur in real-time and often uses email, bulletin board and social networking groups as means for gathering data (see the box below for an example of a study using email interviewing).

There are a number of advantages to gathering data using electronic means. Primarily, there is the potential to recruit a larger and more diverse sample from a wide geographical area without the need to travel. Therefore, time and travel costs are reduced. Where email is used, the cost of and need for transcribing is reduced as the data are already in a written form and is not likely to require significant editing (Meho, 2006). Moreover, the researcher can interview more than one person at a time and the information that is shared is not seen by anybody else (Meho, 2006). Where an asynchronous approach is used participants have the opportunity to reflect and respond in their own time (Meho, 2006). Cook (2012) suggests also that this type of medium is advantageous when recruiting from vulnerable populations as it gives them increased control and comfort. In addition, they may be more likely to make disclosures that they would not do in a face-to-face situation as they are afforded a degree of anonymity. Cook (2012) also argues online interviews may provide a means of accessing potential participants where access by other means, such as through clinicians, is denied.

However, as with all other types of interview there are limitations. While the use of online interviews might capture those who are more comfortable communicating online, this medium excludes those who do not have access or cannot use a computer (Robson, 2011). Synchronous online interviews are limited by time differences and may require either the researcher or the participants to be online at night. Asynchronous interviews may lead to a large number of exchanges between researcher and participant thus taking some considerable time to complete. Also, in online interviews where the discourse is entirely text-based the lack of visual or aural cues can limit ability to achieve a rapport between the researcher and participants (McKeown et al., 2010).

Example of How Email Interviewing was used in a Research study

Title: Email interviewing: generating data with a vulnerable population (Cook, 2012)

Aim of the study: to explore what the diagnosis of a viral sexually transmitted infection (STI) meant to women's lives, the impact on healthcare experiences and their social and sexual lives using a feminist, post-structuralist approach.

Interviews:

- Email advertisement with a link to the university web page detailing the study.
- Designated email address for interviews only.
- 26 women (aged 22–71) from New Zealand, Canada, USA and England with a diagnosis of either human papilloma virus (HPV) or genital herpes simplex virus (HSV).
- 16 interview questions with approximately four questions being emailed at a time (examples below).
  - Similarities or differences in consultation process with health professionals as compared to other conditions
  - Difficulties with asking questions of health professionals
  - Suggestions about the 'ideal' consultation process
  - Any changes in discussing sexuality and sexual health with partner
  - Any changes in the meaning of sexuality.
- Interviews ended after 16 questions with agreement by researcher to email after three months to elicit any additions or make deletions to narrative and evaluate the online process.
- Online access to the research was provided on completion of the study.

ACTIVITY 9.1

Access: Wells, M. (2009) Surveying the experience of living with metastatic breast cancer: comparing face-to-face and online recruitment (paper 578) *Journal of Research in Nursing.* 14: 57–9, through the link below and jot down what you see are the advantages and disadvantages of face-to-face and online recruitment.

http://jrn.sagepub.com/content/14/1/57

Regardless of the approach chosen, undertaking interviews is not an easy option and requires careful planning. Health and social care professionals are used to conducting clinical interviews with people in their care with the result that research interviews are sometimes thought to be quick and easy to conduct. However, research interviewing has a different purpose and is a highly demanding activity and a skill that requires practice. Determining the structure of the interview, having an interview schedule or guide that has been rigorously developed, practise interviewing, deciding the length, timing and number of interviews, and deciding how the data will be recorded, are fundamental elements of preparation. In addition, issues such as access, vulnerability, confidentiality, researcher and participant safety, identification of an appropriate location and determining whether individual, group or online approaches are most appropriate must all be addressed in advance.

Observation

Observation is a data collection strategy that involves the direct observation of phenomena in their natural setting and is used across the spectrum of research methodologies and with varying degrees of structure. For example, it is the foundational method of data collection in ethnographic studies where researchers immerse themselves in the setting to varying degrees, but it is also used by those who are undertaking structured observation using activity or behaviour checklists. Parahoo (2006) states that observation is suited to the study of behaviours such as interaction and performance as well the observation of psychomotor and other non-verbal activities. However, and as outlined in (Chapter 5, box p. 79) observation does not always involve people and can include objects that form part of the setting, events that take place and/or the timing or sequence of those events.

Observation can be used also in studies where it is not possible to collect the information in any other way. For example, potential participants may be unable to participate in interviews or answer questionnaires and where proxy responders may not have sufficient knowledge or data to answer on the participants' behalf (Mansell, 2011). It can be used also to generate research hypotheses where not much is known about the problem. Observation is often used in combination with other strategies such as interviews. This may include on-the-spot conversations that arise from the researcher's observations and where he/she may want to explore why a person behaved or acted in a particular way. In other situations, it may be that formal interviews are conducted to discuss what has been observed but as a discrete and separate activity. These additional data collection methods can add depth and clarity to the observations.

Format of Observation

Four types of observation have been described and include: the complete participant; the participant-as-observer; the observer-as-participant and the complete observer.

Complete Participant

The complete participant is a role whereby the researcher becomes part of the group being observed and engages with the activities of that group (Watson et al., 2010).

Data are collected openly or covertly where the latter can be likened in modern media terms to going 'undercover'. In social research these studies have been justified on the grounds that it would be dangerous to attempt overt study or where it is unlikely that members of the group would willingly participate. While there have been studies in health and social care that have involved covert observation it is highly unlikely in contemporary research that ethical approval would be obtained. Covert observation means that those being observed are not aware of it, have not given their consent and are essentially being deceived.

The Participant-as-observer

The participant-as-observer is the most commonly used role in qualitatively-based observational studies. In this type of observation the researcher becomes part of or works as part of the group under study. The researcher's role is known and informed consent is obtained from all those involved.

The Observer-as-participant

The observer-as-participant is similar to participant-as-observer although in the former the researcher participates only by being in the location rather than working there. Thus, these researchers are not part of the workforce and do not play a 'real' role in the setting.

The Complete Observer

Complete observers are not part of the setting and can be likened to the frequently used 'fly-on-the-wall' approach evident in popular television. Therefore, these researchers have no impact on the situation and have to use strategies such as a two-way mirror or cameras to record what is happening.

While these approaches are presented as discrete entities, in reality there can be crossover particularly between the participant-as-observer and the observer-as-participant modes. For example, researchers may, at the beginning of a study, choose to adopt a primarily observing role but when they become accepted and familiar with the environment they may engage more actively thus moving to more participant-as-observer.

Undertaking Observation

Structured Observation

As indicated above, observations can be structured. Generally, those using structured observations tend to have a non-participant role in that they simply observe and do not engage in the setting. Researchers come to the setting to observe particular activities or behaviours. These activities are broken into discrete units and used to create a checklist. These can be simple such as recording if a healthcare professional washed their hands before and after each patient contact or can be more complex such as observing the hand-washing process. In the latter, a checklist detailing each step of the hand-washing process would have had to be prepared in advance. However, not all structured observations can be as well-defined as the hand-washing process. For example, if researchers wanted to undertake structured observation of challenging behaviour, they would have to clearly define what they meant because there is a risk of differing interpretations.

Unstructured/Qualitative Observation

Studies that use observation can also use what is described as unstructured or qualitative observation. Unstructured observation is normally undertaken in situations where little is known about the phenomenon. The term unstructured implies that researchers may enter a setting with no pre-conceived idea of what they are going to observe. Although it may be the case that they will not have highly developed research questions or objectives, it is very likely that they will, at the very least have identified the phenomenon of interest. For an example of how observation was used in a research study see Lauzon Clabo's (2008) example in the box below.

Example of how Observation was used in a Research Study

An ethnography of pain assessment and the role of social context on two postoperative units (Lauzon Clabo, 2008)

Aim of the study: to examine nursing pain assessment practice across two units.

Research questions:

- In what ways and to what extent does postoperative pain assessment vary across two nursing units?
- What is the impact of nursing unit social context on pain assessment practice?

Observation schedule:

Phase 1:

- Gaining entry (to hospital and two units), establishing relationships with staff, establishing researcher's role.
- Participant observation involved being present in the two units during the course of normal care and interacting informally with staff in hallway conversations in order to become familiar with general routines and to facilitate mapping of the social context (descriptive observation).
- Data recorded using field notes and observational, theoretical and methodological notes.

Phase II:

- Direct observation of 20 day shift nurses as they undertook pain assessment.
- Semi-structured interviews in relation to each assessment.
- Data recorded using field notes.

Note: Focus group interviews were also undertaken in this study and formed Phase III.

As in Lauzon Clabo's study, it is likely that observation will become more focussed as the research progresses. Periods of observation, interacting with those in the setting, writing field notes and reflecting on what is happening facilitates identification of issues that are important because they relate to the research aim. Ultimately, the observation may become highly selective. For example, Lauzon Clabo eventually focussed on observing practitioners as they undertook pain assessment.

Observation is not without its difficulties and demands some of which include: the skills required to undertake observation; gaining access and acceptance by those being observed; clarifying and establishing the observer role; addressing ethical issues about disclosing the focus of the research; deciding what is to be observed; the amount of time needed to undertake observation; and deciding how the observations are to be recorded. As can be reasoned from the points above, observing what is happening in a setting and/or the behaviour of people in that setting is a complex endeavour. Even though observation is a fundamental skill of effective healthcare practitioners, it is nonetheless a difficult task particularly in the descriptive phase at the beginning of a study.

It may be the case also that the role of the researcher and perhaps the ability to be a participant or an observer will be affected if a researcher is not a member of the community or setting being observed. For example, if a social researcher is observing physiotherapists within their own department in a hospital, then their role, insights and understanding will not be the same as if the researcher were a physiotherapist.

Gaining access or entry to the setting and recruiting to studies that use observation can be difficult as practitioners/organisations may not like the idea of others observing their practice. Therefore, even when informed consent has been obtained researchers must allocate sufficient time to enable those who are being studied to get used to being observed and feel comfortable with it.

For researchers, it takes time to become used to the setting and achieve prolonged engagement. In addition, it is almost certain that they will have to re-iterate their role and position and adopt strategies to maintain it. For example, Baumbusch (2011) reported in her critical ethnography in long-term residential care that she was asked by practitioners for feedback on their performances and in other instances was asked to perform nursing duties that were outside the parameters of her researcher role. The difficulty of maintaining an observer status in clinical settings is a known problem in ethnographic studies.

As indicated earlier, it is unlikely that researchers will obtain ethical approval for covert observation in healthcare settings. However, there may be situations where researchers do seek permission to observe but may not reveal the detail of what is being observed. For some, the argument centres on the potential benefit for a greater number of people than it will harm. For example, although it was not healthcare research *per se*, an undercover investigation by a television programme into the care provided in a nursing home in Ireland led to a major outcry about conditions in which the residents lived. As a direct result, the Health Information and Quality Authority (HIQA), (www.hiqa.ie) was established, a move which is seen to have had far-reaching benefits for those in nursing home care. While the results of this particular investigation are persuasive, researchers, Parahoo (2006) suggests, must balance the potential benefits against possible harm when proposing to use any form of concealment. Moreover, unlike investigative journalism researchers are bound by moral and ethical principles that are policed by research ethics committees who will make the ultimate decision about what is and what is not acceptable.

A further issue in observation is deciding what is to be observed. In structured observations this is usually pre-determined but where unstructured or qualitative observation is used it can be less clear, particularly in the descriptive phase. The over-arching premise is that it is not possible to observe everything all the time. Researchers then have to decide who, what, where, when and why they are observing. In this way, they can draw up a schedule for observation. For example, they may undertake periods of observation at different times and on different days so that they can get a picture of what is happening across the whole day. Also, it means that participants in the study are not exposed to constant observation, which could be difficult for them to tolerate. However, even when observation is confined to discrete periods, it is extremely demanding in terms of time needed to complete it.

A strategy is also important because researchers are human and will enter any setting with pre-conceptions (social, cultural, professional), whether they are aware of them or not and may well be influenced by these while observing. Thus, even in structured observations two researchers may classify a behaviour differently. Think of the anecdotes about the wildly different accounts of people who have witnessed the same events. In addition, researchers must be careful not to be intrusive in the setting as this can create what is known as an 'observer effect' (Holloway & Wheeler, 2010). There has been discussion also of the 'Hawthorne' effect where those being observed change their behaviour in response to the presence of the researcher. There appears to be agreement that being observed does change behaviour but the magnitude of the effect and whether this can be sustained over a long period of time remains largely unknown (McCambridge et al., 2014).

Once the observation schedule has been decided another key element is deciding how the observations are to be recorded. If the researcher is a participant in the setting then it is very difficult to make notes. In these instances, researchers often rely on memory and completing field notes as soon as possible after leaving the setting. Those in observer roles (and not participating) may find it easier to make notes but those being observed may not feel comfortable with this. Similarly, the use of video may not be acceptable although it does capture the nuances in practice.

Finally, observation is highly challenging and researchers will often feel undertaking interviews is 'easier'. The time it takes to undertake observation is particularly demanding and it often needs to be conducted in conjunction with other data collection methods. Nonetheless, it does offer insights to practice that are not possible with other methods.

Documentary Sources

Documents are often used in conjunction with other data collection methods but it is possible for a study to be based exclusively on documentary analysis. For example, in historical research, data are often in the form of written records such as published reports, newspapers, diaries and letters. In these situations, documents are used as a means to provide insight into a situation that cannot be directly observed or researched. Documentary sources have been referred to as secondary data because the data were collected (as in a census) or were originally written (as in a diary) for a purpose other than research.

Types of Documents

There are a wide range of documents that are relevant for study within health and social care. As indicated in Table 9.1, these can include documents that are in the public domain, documents with restricted access and published materials.

Documents in the public domain such as autobiographies, biographies, official documents and reports, and media publications can be accessed, for the most part, by anybody at any time. Because they are in the public domain they are not subject to the same access and ethical permissions that would be required of closed or restricted documents. Often there are data contained therein that are of interest to health and social care researchers. This can range from a study of historical records that might offer an explanation for a contemporary or current situation to an analysis of census data to examine health and healthcare trends. Because of this health policy and epidemiological researchers often have a particular interest in documentary data.

Published materials are similar to documents in the public domain in that they can be accessed through libraries or online databases but they may be subject to licensing or subscription restrictions. For example, most universities pay subscriptions to a large number of journals so that staff and students can access materials for their academic studies. Most notably these include reports of research studies, theoretical and discussion papers, and books.

In contemporary health and social care, systematic reviews are a prime example of how previously published research is used in a particular way. Systematic reviews are generally classed as 'research on research' or secondary research as they do not collect new data but use the findings from previous research. In a systematic review the findings of all previous research are pooled and analysed in order to arrive at conclusions about the strength of the evidence that exists on a given topic.

Documents with restricted access, as the name implies, are those that are not in the public domain and for which permission has to be sought in order to access them. This applies, for example, to all clinical documents that relate to the care of patients, clients or users of a service. This is important because even though practitioners have access to these documents for the purposes of providing care to the patient, they cannot be used for any other purpose, such as research, without specific permission to do so. This is a basic principle of data protection, which is concerned with upholding the rights of individuals to have control over their personal data. For example, if a researcher wanted to analyse patient data permission would be needed from the organisation in which the data are stored but also from the patients concerned if that data have not been anonymised. As you can imagine, it can be a difficult task to seek permission from every patient to access their medical records. Therefore, many researchers who seek to use clinical records or documents will only seek permission from the organisation and the appropriate ethics committee to access anonymised data.

When documents are used in research a fundamental aspect is making some determination of their quality. The processes for doing so will vary depending on the type of document used. For example, in systematic reviews, researchers undertake a methodological quality assessment of previous studies. In doing so, they can make a judgement about the veracity and dependability of the findings of each study.

However, other types of documents can be more problematic. Knight (2002) presents the argument that official documents are full of subjectivity. A fundamental question is the credibility of the original author in terms of their intentions, the perspective from which they were writing and whether they were qualified to do so

(Holloway & Wheeler, 2010). Most people are aware, for example, that records of historical events can differ considerably and researchers must attempt to determine if the record they are studying can be regarded as an accurate account. It is necessary also to study the social, political or economic context in which the report was developed and make an interpretation within this context. In addition to recognising the potential biases in published documents, it is also important for researchers to recognise and acknowledge their own assumptions when interpreting such material.

Chapter Summary

This chapter has outlined the most commonly used methods of data collection in healthcare research and included measurement scales, questionnaires, interviews, observation and documentary sources. The characteristics of each were described including the types of data that are collected. Examples, variations, strengths and limitations of each of the methods were outlined.

🔑 Key Points 🔑

- Choosing the most appropriate method of collecting data is fundamental to ensuring the study is credible.
- Data collection is the process used by researchers to collect the necessary information to meet the aim of their study and can involve: the use of measurement scales, questionnaires, interviews, observation and documentary sources.
- Questionnaires, tests and scales are used to measure or test an array of phenomena such as knowledge, attitudes, beliefs, intentions, cognition, functional status, emotion/mood, health status, quality of life and behaviour.
- For the most part questionnaires use forms of closed questions such as two-way, multiple choice, ranking, scaling, contingency, checklist.
- Questionnaires, tests and scales produce different levels of data that are classified as nominal; ordinal; interval; and ratio.
- Interviews can offer insights into the experiences, perceptions or views of people about a particular phenomenon.
- Interviews are broadly classified as structured, semi-structured or unstructured, can be conducted with individuals and in groups, on the telephone or using electronic means.
- Observation is a data collection strategy that involves the direct observation of phenomena in their natural setting and are broadly classified as structured and unstructured.
- Four types of observation have been described: the complete participant; the participant-as-observer; the observer-as-participant and the complete observer.
- Documents are used as a means to provide insight into a situation that cannot be directly observed or researched and are referred to as secondary data.

Useful Online Resources

http://groups.eortc.be/qol/sites/default/files/archives/guidelines_for_developing_
   questionnaire-_final.pdf

10

Gaining Insight into Data Analysis

Introduction

Data analysis is a set of procedures undertaken by researchers to make sense of the data and provide an answer to the research question/hypothesis posed at the beginning of the study. How it is undertaken depends on the type of data that have been collected. Part of reading and understanding research is the ability to comprehend the analytic processes that researchers have applied to their data and grasping how they came to the results they did. Yet, it is not uncommon when reading research reports to be tempted to by-pass the data analysis section and skip straight to the findings of the study. This is because it is the findings that are of most interest but also because many of us find the data analysis section daunting and difficult to understand. Nevertheless, challenging as it may be to unravel and understand how researchers arrive at their findings, it is important as healthcare practitioners that we do so because of the potential implications for our practice. Not only does the data analysis process outline how the researchers managed the data but it provides us with the necessary information to determine if the findings have legitimacy.

Although an in-depth discussion of all the analytical processes available to the modern researcher is beyond the scope of this text, the chapter provides a general overview so that you can engage with and make a judgement about the management of the data in studies you are reading. The chapter presents the characteristics of numerical and narrative analytical processes and outlines situations in which each would be used.

☑ Learning Outcomes ☑

By the end of this chapter you should be able to:

- Outline the purpose of data analysis
- Describe the key characteristics of numerical and narrative data analysis

- Explain the relationship between the type of data and the process of analysis
- Judge if appropriate analytical processes have been applied to the data.

Analysis of Numerical Data

Numerical data (numbers) are managed using a range of statistical procedures that essentially enable organisation, interpretation and communication of information. In other words, statistical procedures are the means by which sense can be made of the data. What researchers want to find out determines the type of numbers they collect, which in turn governs the type of statistical analysis that can be undertaken. These decisions are made in advance of data collection and involve considerable planning to ensure that the data collection tools or instruments that are used gather the required type or level of data.

The first thing you need to know when examining the analysis of data undertaken by researchers is the type of data or level of measurement that has been undertaken. In Chapter 9, (Table 9.3) we outlined the four levels of data (nominal, ordinal, interval, ratio). Often, these are further classified as categorical (nominal and ordinal) and continuous (interval and ratio) (see Figure 10.1). Categorical data, such as nominal and ordinal level are those which can be categorised into distinct groups but have no inherent numerical value. Continuous data, which have numerical value and include interval and ratio level, can be measured along a continuum. When you know the level of data, it can help you decide how to interpret it because the type of data and level of measurement are associated with the type of analysis that can be undertaken. What can be done with each level of data is outlined in Table 10.1.

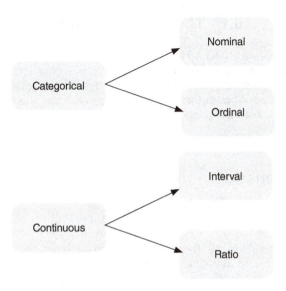

Figure 10.1   Types of quantitative data

Table 10.1　Analysis by level of data (measurement)

Analysis	Nominal	Ordinal	Interval	Ratio
Frequency of Distribution	X	X	X	X
It is possible to 'order' the scores		X	X	X
Mode, median		X	X	X
Mean			X	X
Difference between the scores is quantifiable			X	X
Can add or subtract scores			X	X
Can multiply and divide scores				X
Has an 'absolute zero'				X

ACTIVITY 10.1

Examine the data below and indicate which are nominal, ordinal, interval or ratio. Try to rationalise your decisions. The answers are at the end of the chapter.

1. The birth weight of infants born in one hospital in 2013.
2. Allocation of the numbers 1 and 2 to differentiate males and females who are undertaking a primary degree in healthcare in one university.
3. Level of educational attainment, e.g. A-levels, Primary Degree, Higher Degree.
4. The numbers on the back of jerseys worn by a rugby team.
5. A customer satisfactory survey.
6. Annual income of a group of footballers.
7. The length of hospital stay of patients who were admitted for hip replacements.
8. A health related quality of life tool.
9. Daily temperatures for the month of December.

10.1　Thoughts and Tips

Data on a Likert scale (ranging from strongly disagree to strongly agree) are often allocated numbers, for example, 1–5 or 1–7 for the purposes of analysis. Researchers may then treat these numbers as interval level data assuming equivalence between the points on the scale. While this practice is relatively common, it is not correct and the data should be treated as ordinal.

Descriptive Statistics

Generally, the type of data collected will have the purpose of 'describing' and/or 'inferring'. As the name implies, descriptive statistics tend to be used to describe the characteristics of those involved in a study. They reduce large amounts of data to a more manageable form. What is described will vary depending on the purpose of the study but examples include descriptions of age, gender, presence or absence of a disease, knowledge levels, alcohol and smoking consumption patterns and so on.

The three main features of descriptive statistics that involve analysis of one variable at a time (univariate analysis) are frequency/distribution, central tendency and dispersion/measures of variability.

Descriptive Analysis

Frequency/Distribution

Frequency or distribution is concerned with how many times a value appears in the data. These can be presented as actual numbers, represented by *n*, percentages or if there are large numbers by category. It is worth noting that comparing actual numbers is not always the most accurate representation. For example, in a group of 100 postgraduate students, there are 60 females and 40 males. Forty of the females reported they had a primary degree while 25 of the males did so. These whole numbers cannot be compared as the size of the groups differ. However, when converted to proportions or percentage they offer some insight, that is, 40/60 = 66.6 per cent and 25/40 = 62.5 per cent. Frequency distributions are often represented by tables, bar or pie charts (see Table 10.2 and Figure 10.2).

Table 10.2   Frequency distribution table of diagnoses of participants in a study

Diagnosis	Number (n)
Strokes	10
Respiratory/Circulatory	6
Cancer	4
Alzheimer's Disease	3
Intellectual Disability	2
Parkinson's Disease	1

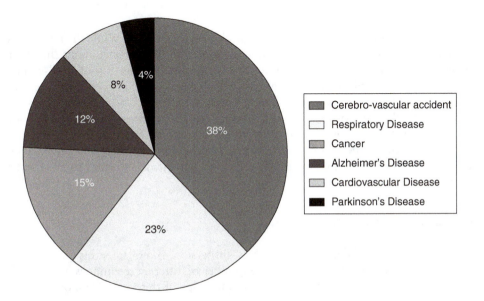

Figure 10.2   Pie chart of diagnoses of participants in a study

Central Tendency

Central tendency is concerned with identifying a single value that best represents the distribution of the data (Robson, 2011). Although statisticians and researchers tend not to use the term 'average' this is essentially what is being sought when using measures of central tendency. There are three measures of central tendency: the mode, the median and the mean.

The mode is the most frequently occurring value and the median is the midpoint when all the scores are arranged in ascending order. The mean more accurately described as the *arithmetic mean* is the average obtained by summing all the scores and dividing by the number of scores available (see the box below).

Calculation of Mode, Median and Mean

Set of scores:

   21, 21, 22, 24, 24, 24, 25, 26, 27 28, 29

Mode: 24 – 24 occurs three times.

Median: 24 – There are 11 scores in total. Therefore, the mid-point is the sixth score (five above and five below). If there is an even number then the two middle scores are selected and divided by two to calculate the median.

Mean (arithmetic mean): Adding all the scores and dividing by 9

$$\frac{21+21+22+24+24+24+25+26+27+28+29}{9}$$

$$= 24.63$$

There are limitations with the use of the mode and the median. While the mode tells us which score occurs most frequently it does not tell us anything about the other scores. There may be extreme scores in the distribution but this cannot be discerned from the mode. Similarly, the median will tell us that 50 per cent of the scores are above and below the median but again it tells us nothing about those scores. In order to calculate an arithmetic mean, the data must be at interval or ratio level. For example, it would be nonsense to calculate an average of data that has no numeric value. While these calculations give us some insight into the dispersion of the data, they are insufficient for making sense of it. Therefore, it is important to have some idea of how the scores vary in a set of data.

Dispersion/Measures of Variability

The third element of descriptive statistics, dispersion, offers some insight into the spread of scores in a dataset. There are a number of different techniques for measuring dispersion or variance that are beyond the scope of this text but an overview is

Table 10.3   Dispersion/measures of variability

Range	Difference between the highest and lowest score
Inter-quartile range	The difference between the 1st and 3rd quartile scores. The 1st quartile is the score that has 25% of the scores **below** it and the 3rd quartile is that which has 25% of the scores **above** it
Variance	The average of the squared deviations (differences) from the mean
Standard Deviation	A calculation of the average deviation (difference) of the scores from the mean. They can be positive or negative OR the square root of the variance
Mean Deviation	A calculation of the average deviation (difference) of the scores from the mean **but** ignoring the signs (positive/negative)

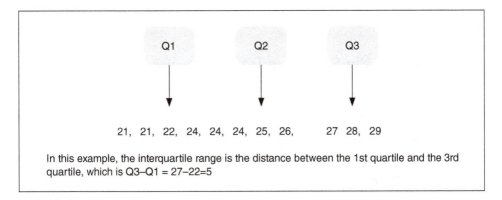

In this example, the interquartile range is the distance between the 1st quartile and the 3rd quartile, which is Q3–Q1 = 27–22=5

Figure 10.3   Interquartile range

presented in Table 10.3. The most commonly cited are the range, the standard deviation and the variance. The range is simply the difference between the highest and lowest scores. Taking our example in the box above, the lowest score is 21 and the highest 29. Therefore, the range is 8, (29–21). The problem is that it only uses two values and is therefore considered unreliable for measuring variability in a data set. In some instances, a measure known as the inter-quartile range may be used as it is considered a better description of the variability in a set of scores. This is because it focuses on scores nearer the centre and excludes possibly extreme scores. It is arrived at by calculating the difference between the first and third quartiles in a set of scores. (Figure 10.3).

Standard Deviation

Standard deviation is probably the most widely used measure of variability with interval or ratio level data. Essentially it calculates the dispersion of the scores in a dataset in relation to the mean. What is important is that it is always used in conjunction with the mean and should be used with interval and ratio data only. It calculates the average difference (deviations) of the scores in the study from the mean and these can be positive or negative. If there is little or no deviation from the mean then the score is close to zero. A worked example is provided in the box below but all contemporary spread-sheet and statistics programs calculate the Standard Deviation. You must remember, however, that the program will calculate any numbers that are entered. Therefore, it is the researcher's responsibility to ensure that the data is either at interval or ratio level of measurement. The formula for standard deviation is presented in Figure 10.4.

$$S = \sqrt{\frac{\Sigma(x - \bar{x})^2}{n-1}}$$

X = each score
$\bar{x}$ = the mean or average
n = the number of values
Σ = the sum of the values

Figure 10.4   Standard deviation

Calculating the Standard Deviation of a Set of Scores

Scores: 21, 21, 22, 24, 24, 24, 25, 26, 27 28, 29

Step 1: Calculate the mean of the scores

21 + 21 + 22 + 24 + 24 + 24 + 25 + 26 + 27 + 28 + 29

11 = 24.63

Step 2: Subtract the mean from each score and square the difference

Score	Difference from mean	Squared result
21	−3.63	13.17
21	−3.63	13.17
22	−2.63	6.91
24	0.63	0.39
24	−0.63	0.39
24	−0.63	0.39
25	0.37	0.13
26	1.37	1.87
27	2.37	5.61
28	3.37	11.35
29	4.37	19.09

Step 3: Work out the averages of the squared difference

13.17 + 13.17 + 6.91 + 0.39 + 0.39 + 0.39 + 0.13 + 1.87 + 5.61 + 11.35 + 19.09

11−1* = 7.24

Note: 7.24 is the variance
*see thoughts and tips

Step 4: Calculate the SD by taking the square root of the variance
$\sigma = \sqrt{7.24} = 2.69$

10.2   Thoughts and Tips

You will notice from the calculation above that the $n - 1$ (number of scores − 1) was used in the calculation of the SD. While most formulae for Standard Deviation have $n-1$, known as Bessel's Correction, there are times when you will simply see n. Either option is available on calculators or in excel. It is said that for an unbiased estimate of the population SD $n - 1$ is used whereas n is appropriate on its own when 'describing' variation in the sample data. Differences in the results tend to be insignificant unless the sample size is small.

So what does the standard deviation tell us? Essentially it tells us the spread of the results and how closely the scores are clustered around the mean. It also allows us to draw some conclusions about those scores but only in the presence of what is known as a *normal distribution* (Bell) or Gaussian curve.

The normal distribution, which tells us about the spread of the data is important as many statistical tests have been developed from the idea that scores are normally distributed. In a normal distribution most of the scores are clustered around the mean (centre) with the frequency of scores falling off at either side. Where there are 'extreme' scores these are more or less distributed evenly above and below the mean (Figure 10.5). In a truly normal distribution, the mode, median and mean are the same and although data rarely follow this pattern exactly, examples of variables that do include height, intelligence and blood pressure. However, what is important for the purpose of illustration here is that when the scores in a dataset are normally distributed the standard deviation enables the following conclusions to be drawn:

- 68 per cent of scores fall within one standard deviation above or below the mean
- 95 per cent scores fall within two standard deviations above or below the mean
- 99 per cent of scores fall within three standard deviations above or below the mean.

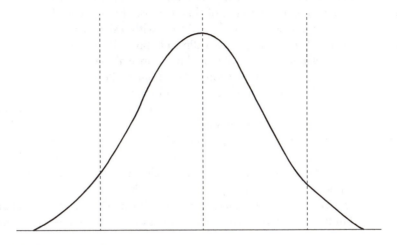

Figure 10.5   Normal distribution curve

As a final point, most publications confine discussion of descriptive analysis to uni-variate (one variable) analysis. However, you may see reference to bivariate (two variables) descriptive statistics, which involves describing the relationship between two variables and is largely associated with correlation research (see Chapter 5). Although these studies can be descriptive whereby the frequency distribution of two variables are cross-tabulated, they are discussed in this text in the inferential statis-tics section. This is because they often attempt to make inferences about the exist-ence and/or strength of a relationship between two variables (calculation of correlation indices).

Inferential Statistics

While descriptive statistics tend to focus on the characteristics of the sample in the study, inferential statistics attempt to establish if there is a relationship between variables. They are concerned with making inferences or predictions about the wider population from which the sample was drawn and assessing the probability that the outcomes of the study are dependable and did not happen by chance. In other words, the statistical tests objectively measure the strength of the evidence against the null hypothesis (Bettany-Saltikov & Whittaker, 2013). Inferential statistics can be applied to experimental, quasi-experimental and non-experimental studies and can focus on two (bivariate) or more (multivariate) variables. In the former, the aim is to establish causality (cause and effect) whereas in the latter the purpose may be to simply establish an association or the strength of an association between the variables. Choosing the correct inferential test therefore depends on the research hypothesis and the type (level) of data that are gathered.

Significance Level/Probability

Researchers can never be 100 per cent certain that the findings of their studies are true and did not occur by chance. Because of this they use the concept of probability (p), which is expressed on a scale ranging from 0 to 1, with 0 signifying there is no chance of its occurrence and 1 indicating it is certain to happen. Probability is defined as the likelihood that the results were not obtained by chance alone if the null hypothesis is true (Freeman & Walters, 2010; Robson, 2011; Polit & Beck, 2012). The p value is calculated based on the assumption that the null hypothesis is true and tells research-ers how rarely they would observe a difference as large (or larger) than the one they did if the null hypothesis were true. For example, if a null hypothesis states that there is no difference in the pain scores of patients who receive one type of analgesia over another, the p value specifies how closely the results of the study match the null hypothesis. A high p value means there is a higher chance of the result being consistent with the null hypothesis, while a low p value means the probability is lower.

Therefore, statistical testing is undertaken to establish how likely it is that any dif-ference is attributable to the independent variable rather than chance. If it is unlikely that the difference was caused by chance then the results are seen as significant. Essentially, this is the level at which the researcher is prepared to accept or reject the null hypothesis. What is deemed to be significant is a matter of convention and is usually set at 1/20 or 0.05 (Robson, 2011). It is usually expressed as a probability value and represented as $p \leq 0.05$ although in certain situations a smaller p value may be set, for example, $p \leq 0.01$.

Research Hypothesis

Studies that are concerned with making inferences begin with a research hypothesis (see Chapter 3) that is tested. Simply stated, if there is no hypothesis then there is no statistical test. As indicated in Chapter 3, a research hypothesis comprises a statement that makes some prediction of the outcome of the study. The prediction may focus on examining associations between variables or seeking differences. For example, the hypothesis that the amount of processed food ingested daily has an effect on children's weight can be answered in a number of ways. For instance, the researcher might seek to establish if there is a relationship between the variables and how strong it is through a correlational design while in an experimental study, he/she might examine the differences in weight gain in children related to processed food intake. The point here is that the research design, its subsequent measures (data collection tools) and level of data indicate what statistical tests are undertaken.

Type (Level) of Data

There are two main classifications of inferential tests: parametric and non-parametric and it is important to select the correct type based on the criteria for each. Parametric tests are seen to be more sensitive and produce more powerful results than non-parametric tests. The conditions for using parametric tests are outlined in the box below. The most important of these are the first and second and these should not be violated while the third and fourth may not be met in certain conditions. Non-parametric tests can be used with any level of data (nominal, ordinal, interval, ratio).

Conditions for Parametric Tests

1. Interval or ratio level data
2. Normal distribution
3. Subjects should have been randomly assigned
4. Homogeneity of variance (the spread of the two sets of the scores should be similar). Some tests require variances in the population to be similar.

10.3   Thoughts and Tips

The reason that the level of data should be interval or ratio for parametric tests is that they often use the 'mean' as a basis for conducting it. As you will know from earlier you can only calculate the mean with interval or ratio data. For example, the independent *t* test outlined in Table 10.6 analyses the difference between the mean values of two groups while Analysis of Variance (ANOVA) (Table 10.7 and 10.8) examines the mean values of two or more samples, one or more independent variables (IV) and/or two or more conditions.

When reading research reports the first thing to establish is if the study meets the conditions for parametric tests. If not, then you should expect to see that non-parametric tests have been used. However, even if you establish this, there are a large number of parametric and non-parametric tests and it can be quite confusing trying to discern if researchers have chosen the correct ones. Moreover, there are additional considerations that must be taken into account and these relate to the aim of the study, the sample and the number (bivariate or multivariate) of variables or conditions being tested. Table 10.4 outlines these further.

Table 10.4   Choosing a statistical test

Aim of the study	Is the study a test of difference? Is the study a test of relationships?
Type of sample	• One-sample designs One sample only with the results being compared with known properties (mean/standard deviation) of a wider population, e.g. height of individuals in the study compared with the average height of individuals in the wider population • Two-sample designs **Related** • Are the subjects the same, e.g. pre-/post-test (before and after)? • Are the subjects matched (different subjects who are very similar on the variables that might influence the behaviour being studied)? **Independent** • Are the subjects independent (two or more separate groups)?
Number of conditions or variables	Are two conditions being tested? Are more than two conditions being tested?

Table 10.5   Statistical tests for one-sample research designs

Parametric tests	one-sample Z one-sample *t*
Non-parametric tests	One-sample proportions test

Although it is beyond the scope of this text to discuss the details of the tests used, Tables 10.5, 10.6, 10.7, 10.8 and 10.9 present the type of tests you would expect to see depending on the type of data, the number of samples, the number of independent variables and the number of conditions being studied.

10.4 Thoughts and Tips

A 1 sample Z test requires a large sample of n = >30 or the standard deviation of the scores in the **population** must be known. The one sample t test is used in all other conditions. The one sample proportions test uses proportions instead of means because the data is usually at nominal level.

Table 10.6   Statistical tests for two-sample research designs, one independent variable and/or two or more conditions

	Related Samples (same and matched)	Independent Samples
Parametric tests	Related t-test	Independent Z-test Independent t-test
Non-parametric tests	Wilcoxin signed-rank test	Mann-Whitney U test Chi-square (X^2) test

---

10.5 Thoughts and Tips

Conditions generally refer to exposure to the independent variable, e.g. being tested before (condition 1) and after (condition 2) exposure.

10.6 Thoughts and Tips

Chi-square is only used when the level of measurement is nominal and a sample size of at least 20 is needed in each group (otherwise a Fischer's exact test is used).

Table 10.7   Statistical tests for three-sample research designs, one independent variable and/or three or more conditions

	Related Samples	Independent Groups
Parametric tests	One-way Analysis of Variance (ANOVA) (related)	One-way Analysis of Variance (ANOVA) (un-related)
Non-parametric tests	Friedman test	Kruskal-Wallis test

Table 10.8   Statistical tests for two or more independent variables (IV)

	Related Samples*	Independent Groups*
Parametric tests	Two-way repeated measures Analysis of Variance (ANOVA)	Two-way independent measures of Analysis of Variance (ANOVA)
Non-parametric tests		Chi-square (X²) test

*See 10.7 – Thoughts and Tips

10.7   Thoughts and Tips

In some cases one of the independent variables may be an independent measure, for example, three different groups exposed to different treatments while the other is a repeated measure, for example, the same participants in each of the three groups are tested over time. In this instance, a two-way mixed measures Analysis of Variance (ANOVA) is used (Bettany-Saltikov & Whittaker, 2013).

As outlined in Chapter 5, data in correlational studies are visually represented using a 'scattergram' (see Figure 5.3). Ultimately, the relationships between the variables are classified as 'linear', 'non-linear' or 'uncorrelated'. Levels of correlation range from a perfect negative correlation (negative linear relationship) represented as −1.0 to a perfect positive correlation (positive linear relationship) signified as 1.0, with 0.0 indicating no relationship (uncorrelated) as outlined in Figure 10.6. These numbers are known as the 'correlation co-efficient', which is represented as r. A positive correlation (or direct relationship) means the two variables move in the same direction while a negative correlation (or inverse relationship) means the two variables move in opposite directions.

Table 10.9   Statistical tests for correlational research

Parametric tests	Pearson product moment correlation coefficient test (Pearson's r)
Non-parametric tests	Spearman rank order correlation coefficient (Spearman's rho)

While this is the standard method for analysing the strength of an association between two variables, in predictive studies a process known as 'regression' is used. This is because the analysis is not just focussed on the strength of an association but is concerned with determining if the value of one variable, for example, weight can predict the value of another, for instance, blood glucose. Where there is more than one possible explanation influencing the outcome, such as the impact of family history on the development of type 2 diabetes, the process adopted is known as 'multiple regression'.

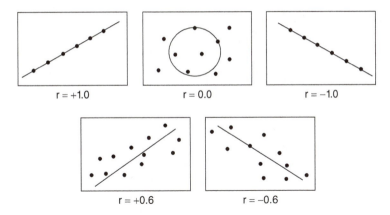

Figure 10.6   Correlational Relationships

Analysis of Narrative (words)

Analysis of narrative or words is frequently referred to as qualitative data analysis. The process usually involves a systematic approach through the use of an identified framework for analysis. Similar to analysis of numbers, the type of analysis that is undertaken is directly related to the purpose of the research study and not all studies take the same approach. Methodologies such as grounded theory, phenomenology and ethnography have distinct ways of analysing data in order to achieve the overall outcome (Holloway & Wheeler, 2010). For example, if the purpose of a study is to *describe* a phenomenon as may be the case in a qualitative descriptive study the approach to analysis will be different to that of a grounded theory study where the purpose is to *develop a theory*. Therefore, the interpretation in a grounded theory study goes beyond description and seeks to explain what may be happening. The intended outcome will direct the type of analytical framework that is chosen. Therefore, when reading studies you should seek to determine researchers' rationale for their approach to analysis and determine if it is most suitable for the purpose of the study.

While qualitative studies differ in their purpose and thereby in their approach to analysis there are some common features and these form the focus of this section. While it is beyond the scope of this text to explore distinct approaches, a generic data analysis framework is presented to demonstrate how these common features can be incorporated into the process.

Data reduction is a universal feature of qualitative data analysis whereby codes and themes and/or categories are created to represent the data. This is because these studies are likely to collect large amounts of data. An hour's interview with a participant can generate up to 10,000 words and field notes and observations can be substantial. Since it is neither practical nor feasible to include all transcripts and field notes in a report or to expect readers to read them, the data is reduced, interpreted and presented in a meaningful way to the reader.

Coming to a meaningful interpretation involves judgements on the part of the researcher and as Ellis (2010) suggests involves the reader trusting that the researcher has remained true to the data. In order to achieve this, researchers adopt a number of strategies (see Chapter 8) but a central feature is reflexivity or critical reflection. As indicated in Chapter 5, the researcher is engaged in the research and in order to ensure that he/she does not unduly influence it, critical reflection is undertaken that may involve acknowledging previous experience and influences, one's own role in the research as well as considering thoughts, feelings and responses to the participants in the study.

Another common feature of qualitative studies is that data collection and data analysis can happen simultaneously whereby data from one wave of data collection are analysed and inform subsequent data collection. This process is referred to as *iteration* and is in contrast to studies that collect numbers whereby data analysis occurs after data collection has been completed.

There are a number of generic data analysis tools that essentially follow the steps of:

- Organising the data
- Becoming immersed in the data
- Reducing the data through coding, identifying themes and/or categories
- Relating the themes and/or categories
- Presenting the outcome.

Organising the Data

Researchers should always indicate how they handled the raw data in preparation for analysis. If their data were in the form of audio-taped interviews then they should indicate if they were transcribed to a written or typed format. While this was always the case in the past the advent of data management systems means that audio material can be imported directly into computerised data management systems. If field notes were gathered as part of observations, they should indicate how these were completed. Although photographic or visual representations of phenomenon are not transformed in any way they may be compiled chronologically or aligned with individual participants.

Other tasks associated with organising the data include ensuring that the raw data are anonymised and all identifiers removed. Researchers usually label transcripts with a pseudonym or code numbers and in their reports make reference to such strategies.

Becoming Immersed in the Data

All data analysis strategies recommend that reading and re-reading of the transcriptions, field notes or other records, possibly in conjunction with listening to audio recordings facilitates immersion in the data. This is regarded as a useful task as it enables the researcher to get a general sense of what the data are saying.

Reducing the Data

Reducing the data is the process of coding, identifying themes and/or categories. Usually, this begins with coding, which is the process of applying descriptive labels that capture what is being said. This can be done manually or using a computer package. A descriptive code, also known as an *invivo* code is the simplest form and it remains close to the terms the participant has used. Coding is not easy and in the initial stages researchers may struggle to arrive at labels they feel best describe what has been said. In order to understand this better, examine the quote in the box below, and apply a label(s) that you feel would describe it most appropriately.

Coding

'If someone has made an effort to come and be in contact with you and listen to what you are saying it adds value to you, because you are worth that effort, aren't you? If you don't feel supported then you don't feel that anyone is listening to you...'

Labels you may have thought of might have been 'feeling supported' and 'being valued' but you probably would have liked to have seen what text came before and after this quote and the context or situation in which the words were spoken. This is a particular difficulty when a process of 'line by line' coding is adopted because researchers may feel they are losing the overall sense what is being said. To counter this, they have to decide how extensive the phrase must be in order to accurately capture its meaning. What this means is that the *unit of analysis* can vary from a single word to a whole paragraph. Usually, researchers will use memos in the margins of the transcript and notes to record decisions they have made at this stage.

10.8 Thoughts and Tips

The process of labelling always involves a level of interpretation. Think of when you are reporting a dialogue you have had to a third person. Unless you use verbatim quotes you will report your summarised interpretation of that dialogue. Similarly, even when a study is deemed to be descriptive and/or speaks of findings that are 'data near', the researcher is still presenting an interpretation.

The process of managing the coding of transcripts will vary from researcher to researcher. Many researchers code directly from the data and this is known as *inductive* coding. In other situations, the first transcript is coded inductively and a template (of codes) is created. This template is then used as a basis for coding subsequent tran-scripts and is adjusted as additional codes are added. It is also possible to use a process known as *apriori* coding. This is where the researcher creates a template of possible codes before the formal analysis process begins. These codes can be derived from the literature or previous research on the topic. This can be advantageous as it reduces the demands of labelling through inductive coding. In addition, it means that the research is already linked to work that has been done before. A fundamental point, however, is that this list of codes must not be considered definitive and data that does not 'fit' must be used to create additional codes and modification of the template.

At this point, the researcher may have a very large number of codes, which can then be re-examined to ensure the labelling is consistent and the best label has been applied. This often results in a reduction in the number of codes. Once this has been completed, the researcher begins the process of grouping similar codes together to create themes or categories (see Figure 10.7). These often constitute the major findings of the study and may be used as the structure for the presentation of findings (Creswell, 2009).

Being able to demonstrate how a label was arrived at for a section of raw data is a key element of demonstrating the rigour or quality of a study. Therefore, it is essential that researchers devise strategies for ensuring they can always link a code/theme to the raw data from which it came. This is particularly the case if the data is being analysed manually. In addition, it is an expectation that when the findings are being discussed that they are illustrated with quotes from the raw data. For a more extensive discussion of qualitative data analysis techniques see: Creswell (2009); Bazely (2013); Moule and Goodman (2014).

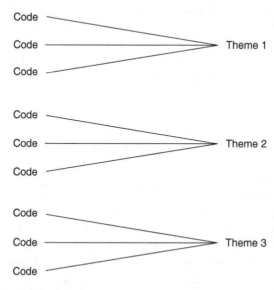

Figure 10.7   Codes and themes

Relating the Themes and/or Categories

At this stage, the researcher will have completed the coding and identified themes and/or categories that represent the raw data. The next step involves determining how these codes and themes are interrelated. So not only are codes related to themes as identified in Figure 10.7 but the themes must be related to each other. This inter-relationship is important in arriving at an overall sense of the phenomenon (the 'whole') that has been the subject of study. The final interpretation is often represented diagrammatically and supported with textual description/explanation. Depending on the purpose of the study it can take various forms such as a description, a narrative, a theory or an ethnograph.

10.9 Thoughts and Tips

The process of analysis has been presented as linear but in reality it is iterative, that is, it moves back and forth between each stage. This is because as the researcher progresses through the analysis he/she may re-visit earlier stages in order to clarify, re-organise or re-define what has gone before.

Presenting the Outcome

Once the analysis is complete the outcome must be presented. This involves presenting the findings and is usually structured using each of the major themes and the codes therein. A fundamental part of this involves including quotes from the raw data to illustrate and justify the classification of codes and themes. There needs to be sufficient detail to enable the reader to make a judgement about the believability of the outcome. It is also about making the data analysis process transparent and is a key part of demonstrating the rigour of the study.

Once the outcome has been presented, the researcher engages in a discussion of the findings in the context of previous research and theories. This is a central part of any study because it enables the researcher to situate his/her study within existing knowledge about the topic. It can include a discussion of where the findings confirm or depart from previous research and theories. Where findings differ, it can involve speculation or a tentative explanation as to why this is the case and will also include suggestions for future studies. Researchers may also explore the implications of the findings of their studies for clinical practice. However, you should remember that in studies that analyse words, these implications are usually confined to the setting and participants in which the research took place. It is not the intention of these researchers to make generalisations outside the study setting but in many instances to provide insight or a new understanding of a phenomenon.

Chapter Summary

This chapter has presented an introduction to data analysis procedures for studies that collect numbers and those that collect words. Although it was beyond the scope of the text to present all analytical procedures the chapter provided a general overview to enable you to engage with and make a judgement about the management of the data in studies you are reading.

A final point is that the findings of all studies remain open and results must be interpreted with caution. It would be rare to implement changes in clinical practice on the basis of the findings of one study. This 'rule' applies to all types of studies. Studies that are qualitatively based acknowledge their subjectivity and do not make claims to be representative of a wider population but there is a risk in quantitative studies that statistically significant findings can be interpreted as 'proof'. However, this is not the case and they are open to further proof or even being disproved.

🔑 Key Points 🔑

- Data analysis is a set of procedures undertaken to make sense of the data and provide answers to research questions/hypotheses.
- Numerical data are managed using a range of statistical procedures in order to make sense of the data.
- The type of statistical analysis is governed by the level of data that are collected.
- Descriptive statistics are used to describe the characteristics of those involved in a study. The three main features in univariate analysis are frequency/distribution, central tendency and dispersion/measures of variability.
- Inferential statistics are concerned with making inferences or predictions about the wider population from which the sample was drawn and assessing the probability that the outcomes of the study are dependable and did not happen by chance. Inferential statistics focus on bivariate or multivariate analysis.
- Probability is defined as the likelihood that the results were not obtained by chance alone if the null hypothesis is true.
- There are two main classifications of inferential tests: parametric and non-parametric.
- Analysis of narrative or words is frequently referred to as qualitative data analysis in the literature. Not all studies take the same approach. Methodologies such as grounded theory, phenomenology and ethnography have distinct ways of analysing data.
- The steps/stages of qualitative data analysis commonly include: Organising; Immersing; Reducing; Relating and Presenting the data.

---

1. Ratio: Weight is measured at equivalent intervals and there is an absolute zero. There is no such thing as a minus weight.
2. Nominal: This is simply the allocation of a number to differentiate between males and females (gender).
3. Ordinal: There is a suggested order but the intervals between them are not the same.
4. Nominal: The numbers are simply identifying the position of a player, they do not have any numerical value.
5. Ordinal: Responses are likely to be on a scale which is given a number. However, the interval between the numbers is not equal.
6. Ratio: Money is ratio data because the intervals between the numbers is equal and there is an absolute zero.

7. Ratio: Length of hospital stay is measured in days, which are of equal interval and there is an absolute zero.
8. Ordinal: Options on a health-related quality of life tool may be given a number but the interval between them is not equal.
9. Interval: The interval between temperatures is equal but there is no absolute zero. It is possible to have minus temperatures.

Useful Online Resource

http://cast.massey.ac.nz/

11

How is Research Disseminated and Implemented?

Introduction

> Communicating research findings, the final step of the research process, involves developing a research report and disseminating it through presentation and publication. (Burns & Grove, 2005: 585)

In considering the above sentence, it is important for you to understand that the research process cannot be considered complete until such a time as the findings have been written-up, reported and disseminated. Not only is it unethical to conduct research and not report the findings but it is disadvantageous to clinical practice and healthcare progress. Indeed, funding bodies, government departments and/or healthcare institutions invariably require researchers to document a detailed dissemination plan prior to undertaking a research study. The focus of this chapter is to explore and discuss research dissemination and implementation. Essential criteria for reporting and dissemination are discussed and strategies for disseminating research are explored. The importance of disseminating research findings and their implications for future study will be addressed. Lastly, the barriers and facilitators to research implementation will be explored.

☑ Learning Outcomes ☑

At the end of this chapter you should be able to:

- Understand essential criteria in research dissemination
- Describe the various strategies that can be used for research dissemination
- Describe the importance of research dissemination

- Understand the implications of research findings for future studies
- Discuss the barriers and facilitators to research implementation.

Essential Criteria in Research Reporting and Dissemination

As research findings can impact on what we do in clinical practice and how we do it, dissemination of research findings brings with it a degree of responsibility. Researchers must accept this responsibility, and, in doing so, adhere to the essential criteria of accurate reporting, truthfulness and credibility in research dissemination.

Accurate Reporting

History has revealed that inaccurate reporting, misreporting or non-reporting of research does occur and that this can have a significant impact on clinical healthcare. In his book, *Bad Pharma*, Ben Goldacre provides numerous examples of research that has gone unreported, particularly in relation to negative (unfavourable) results in drug studies, and discusses the impact this can have on clinical care (Goldacre, 2012). One such described example relates to an anti-depressant drug called Reboxetine. A relatively small study, conducted on 254 individuals, showed positive results for this drug in treating depression. The results of this study were published in an academic journal for doctors and healthcare users to read. In 2010, a group of researchers searched for and brought together all of the evidence from studies that examined the effectiveness of this drug. What they found were seven studies, six of which were not published, and in which it was found that there was no difference in Reboxetine compared to a placebo in treating depression (Goldacre, 2012). The real issue here is that the findings from these six other studies were not made known to clinicians or to the public. This in turn may have misled doctors to prescribe Reboxetine, thinking it was effective for treating depression when in reality it was not any more effective than a placebo in the majority of instances. The clinical impact of not reporting important results simply because they are not seen to be favourable, is that individuals may go untreated or are treated inappropriately.

In contrast, full reporting of research results can have a profound effect on improving health outcomes. For example, starting in 1972, seven trials were conducted to evaluate whether giving steroids to help mature the baby's lungs in women with signs of preterm labour increases the chances of the baby surviving. Two trials showed significant benefits, that is, steroids saved babies' lives. Five of the trials showed no significant benefit for giving steroids. Arguably this creates a clinical dilemma as the evidence is conflicting. Following the publication of these individual studies, a researcher was able to perform a meta-analysis (a statistical pooling of the results from all of the individual studies). By doing this, it was found that giving steroids to women in preterm labour reduces the risk of baby death by 30 per cent–50 per cent (Crowley, 2006). This significantly changed practice in this area and all women presenting with signs of preterm labour, to this day, are administered prophylactic corticosteroids in an effort to help the baby survive should he/she be born prematurely.

Accurate reporting, not only involves reporting of all studies and their results to the wider public, but also full disclosure of any limitations associated with a study. Most researchers face some challenges when designing and conducting a study, which can limit the research in some way. This is not usually a problem unless the limitations are very severe. A problem occurs, however, where researchers fail to transparently report these. This is because the readers are denied the opportunity to consider these limitations when considering the strength and usefulness of the results. In this sense, researchers have a responsibility to describe any limitations to their study that might impact on results when disseminating their findings. The box below provides an example of how authors might do this using the published OSCE study example described previously in Chapter 8.

Example of Described 'Limitations' in a Published Study

A number of study limitations, however, must be acknowledged and considered when interpreting the results of this study. Firstly, this study was conducted three months after the OSCE as students were on college holidays ... Students' recall of the OSCE may have faded during that time. Secondly, as students were on clinical placements in the 3 weeks preceding the OSCE assessment, some students may have undertaken clinical placements that provided them with increased lactation and infant feeding practical experience ... (Muldoon et al., 2014: 472)

ACTIVITY 11.1

As an activity, identify a paper reporting a research study on a topic of interest to you. Identify whether the authors have described limitations to their study in the paper. Ask yourself whether their description is sufficient or not. Where the authors have not described limitations, evaluate the study to see if you can identify limitations and ask yourself if these, in turn, impact on the overall results. Where limitations have been described, explore these to determine whether you think there may be further limitations that have not been described. List these and consider how these might impact on using the findings in clinical practice.

Truthfulness

Truthfulness refers to honesty and transparency in reporting research findings and should be considered an essential criterion in research dissemination. You may be thinking that this goes without saying, but as with accurate reporting, history provides us with numerous examples of dishonesty in research dissemination. One such example that some of you may be familiar with, is the controversial claims that the MMR (measles, mumps and rubella) vaccine was harmful. In February 1998, a group led by Andrew Wakefield published a paper in the respected British medical journal, the *Lancet* (Wakefield et al., 1998). The paper implied a link between the MMR vaccine and a 'new syndrome' of autism and bowel disease. Critics, however, pointed out that the paper was based on a small series of cases (12 children) and relied on parental recall and beliefs (Payne & Mason, 1998). Furthermore, numerous subsequent epidemiological studies consistently found no evidence of a link between autism and the MMR vaccine (Godlee et al., 2011). In the wake of the controversy that followed, the General Medical Council (GMC) launched an investigation into the research and its claims. The GMC found that the research was scientifically and ethically flawed with evidence of falsification of data (Godlee et al., 2011). The GMC investigation resulted in the research being retracted and Dr Wakefield being stripped of his clinical and academic credentials (Godlee et al., 2011). Nonetheless, the publication of this research had significant implications for public health. MMR vaccination compliance dropped sharply in the UK, from 92 per cent to 84 per cent between 1996 and 2002 and was as low as 61 per cent in 2003 in some parts of London (Murch, 2009). After vaccination rates dropped, the incidence of measles and mumps increased in the UK. In 1998, for example, there were 56 confirmed cases of measles. This figure rose to 449 in the first five months of 2006, with the first death occurring since 1992 (Asaria & MacMahon, 2006). The incidence of mumps cases began rising also after years of very few cases. By 2005 the UK was in a mumps epidemic with almost 5000 notifications in the first month of 2005 alone (Gupta et al., 2005). This demonstrates the effect that research findings can have on public opinion. The legacy of the MMR vaccine controversy still remains and it may be some years yet, if at all, that public confidence in the vaccine is fully restored.

Credibility

A final essential criterion in disseminating research is researcher credibility. Almost all journals now require authors to provide their qualification credentials and institutional affiliation when submitting their manuscripts for potential publication. You may be wondering what this has to do with research findings. However, disclosure of researcher credentials allows for transparency where readers of the research can assess the qualification levels of those publishing the research. Unqualified or inadequately trained researchers, due to inexperience or a lack of knowledge, potentially could design and conduct research that is of a lesser quality than those more experienced in the field. This, in turn, will compromise the overall results of the study. A highly publicised example of this involved the nutritionist and health guru, Gillian McKeith. Ms McKeith was using the title 'Dr' on the basis of a PhD from an American college. There were public and academic concerns over allegedly inaccurate research claims made by Miss McKeith and her PhD qualification was called into question. As it transpired, Ms McKeith's PhD was attained from a non-accredited institution (Goldacre, 2008). In the wake of this criticism, Ms McKeith withdrew the 'Dr' title from her name (Clout, 2007).

11.1 Thoughts and Tips

When reading research reports it is important to become familiar with examining the researchers'/authors' credentials. In this way, you will begin to think about the researchers, their qualifications and thus their ability to undertake the research study. These details are usually provided directly after the authors name, for example,

(Continued)

(Continued)

Nigel Lee, RM MMid (Midwife/PhD Candidate)[a,d,*], Joan Webster, RN BA (Professor)[b,f], Michael Beckmann, MBBS FRANZCOG (Director of Obstetrics)[c,e], Kristen Gibbons, BMAths(Hons) BinfoTech (Senior Statiscian)[c], Tric Smith, RM MN (Maternity Unit Manager)[b], Helen Stapleton RM PhD (Senior Research Fellow)[a,d], Sue Kildea, BH1thSc (Hons) PhD (Professor of Midwifery)[a,d]

or separately in a paragraph at either the beginning or at the end of the paper.

Amita A. Mahendru[a], Christoph C. Lees[b,*]

[a] *Clinical Research Fellow in Fetal Medicine, Rosie Maternity-Addenbrooke's Hospital, Cambridge University Hospitals NHS Foundation Trust, Hills Road, Cambridge CB2 2QQ, UK*
[b] *Consultant in Obstetrics and Fetal-Maternal Medicine, Rosie Maternity-Addenbrooke's Hospital, Cambridge University Hospitals NHS Foundation Trust, Hills Road, Cambridge CB2 2QQ, UK*

Strategies for Reporting and Dissemination

There are numerous strategies available to disseminate research findings. As students undertaking research modules, you will likely be most familiar with research studies that are published in healthcare journals, and, agreeably, this appears to be the most common method used to report and disseminate research findings. However, it is important to recognise the multiple strategies that can be used for research dissemination and acknowledge the various merits that each one has (Table 11.1). Furthermore, in choosing a strategy, consideration of the target audience is necessary. In this sense, the researcher might ask him/herself who will benefit most from knowing the findings or to whom might the findings be most important. Based on this, the researcher will consider the most appropriate strategy (or strategies) to target this audience. For example, if a researcher wished to communicate findings to users of healthcare, developing flyers, brochures or posters might be beneficial. Flyers, posters and/or brochures can offer a concise and visually appealing way to disseminate information to broad audiences. If the target audience happens to be healthcare professionals in practice, the use of seminars, conferences or journal clubs might provide a better approach for disseminating to these groups. Academics or policy makers, on the other hand, who have access to university libraries, may primarily source information through journal publications, academic theses and/or key textbooks. Researchers should endeavour to disseminate their findings through these means to reach these audiences.

Table 11.1 provides examples of strategies for disseminating research findings. The primary target audiences and some advantages and disadvantages of each type are also provided.

Table 11.1   Strategies for disseminating research

Strategy	Primary target audiences	Advantages	Disadvantages
Healthcare journals, books and theses	Academics, policy makers and practitioners	• Usually peer-reviewed or edited which adds to quality in reporting. • Numerous texts available. • Discipline specific in many cases. • Electronic versions usually available.	• Submission and publication process can be lengthy. • Language usually very scientific. • Subscription for many journals or access to academic library necessary.
Research conferences, seminars, professional meetings, etc.	Academics, professionals and practitioners	• Large audiences. • Allows for face-to-face discussions. • Findings from a number of studies can be presented at one time.	• Time-restricted (i.e. presentations often short). • Can be costly to attend (e.g. conference fee). • Time and resource commitments (venue, time to attend, etc.).
Posters, flyers, brochures, newsletters, etc.	Public and healthcare practitioners	• Wide audience, especially useful for disseminating widely to the public. • Rapid dissemination. • Particularly suitable for presenting graphs and tables. • Visually appealing way of presenting research results.	• Requires extensive simplification of information due to limited space. • Can be costly to produce depending on format and amount.
Government or healthcare organisations' reports	Public, academics, policy-makers, professionals, practitioners and students of healthcare	• In-depth reports. • Freely available, in the main, on Department websites. • Generally detail healthcare matters of particular public interest.	• Can be lengthy and time-consuming to read. • Can be written in such a way that they are not always easily understood by a 'lay-person'. • May have to pay to access some reports.
Healthcare websites/web-postings	Public	• Wide and rapid dissemination (internationally accessible). • Inexpensive/free.	• Source of information not always reliable or accurate.
Other media (radio, television, newspapers, magazines, etc.)	Public	• Wide and rapid dissemination.	• Reports often short with full details not available (reader unable to evaluate conduct of study and thus level of quality of results).

Using Healthcare Journals for Research Dissemination

As students of healthcare you are likely to frequently use journals to access research information to inform academic assignments, clinical practice and other work. For this reason, it is worth exploring journal publication a little further so that you may gain insight into what is involved here.

Choosing the Journal

There are currently hundreds of healthcare journals from which to choose for disseminating research results. For example, as of March 2014, 5669 healthcare journals were indexed for MEDLINE. Many journals are subject or discipline specific. For example, the *Cochrane Database of Systematic Reviews*, in the Cochrane Library, is specific to systematic review publications only. *The Lancet*, a high quality medical and allied healthcare journal, in addition to publishing articles of general medical and healthcare interest, has specialty journals in the fields of global health, diabetes and endocrinology, oncology, neurology, respiratory medicine, and infectious diseases. The journals of *Midwifery* and *Evidence Based Midwifery* will consider research and reports specific to the discipline of maternity care. Similarly there are a number of speciality nursing journals, for example, the *Journal of Trauma Nursing, Surgical and Vascular Nursing, Journal of the American Psychiatric Nurses Association, Geriatric Nursing* and the *Journal of Wound, Ostomy and Continence Nursing*, to name but a few. Submission of a paper to a healthcare journal, in almost all cases, involves an online submission process with the varied journals providing specific guidance to authors.

Journals and their publications can be categorised into two broad types: i) open access; and ii) subscription only. Open access journals are available freely online for all to view. One example of an open access publisher is BioMed Central (BMC). BMC publishes a number of journals across various healthcare disciplines (e.g. BMC Pregnancy and Childbirth, BMC Cancer, BMC Complementary and Alternative Medicine, BMC Family Practice, BMC Emergency Medicine, and many more). Open access publishing allows dissemination to a wide audience who have access to the internet. It also aims for rapid publishing comparative to other journals (e.g. six weeks in some instances). A disadvantage of open access publishing is that it can be costly to the researchers/authors who must pay a fee to have their paper published in an open access journal. This can be as much as 1000–1200 Euros/GBP depending on the journal. The alternative involves subscribing to a journal and paying an annual or monthly fee. Many university libraries will subscribe to journals that are popular and relevant to their courses/disciplines to facilitate students and staff having access to these. Alternatively, you can personally subscribe to a journal of interest to you.

11.2   Thoughts and Tips

Should you feel that there is a journal of particular high relevance to the course you are undertaking and it is not available in your university library, it would be worth speaking to your librarian or your course administrator to determine if this journal might be made available for your course.

Journal Impact Factor

The Impact Factor (IF) of an academic journal is a measure that reflects the frequency with which a journal's articles are cited in the scientific literature (Saha et al., 2003). It is often used as proxy measure for the relative importance of a journal within its field, with journals that have higher IFs deemed more important than those with lower IFs (Polit & Northam, 2011). The IF is calculated based on citation data from the previous two years indexed in the Thomson Reuters Journal Citation Reports, for example. The box below provides a worked example of an IF calculation for 2008.

IF Calculation

A = The number of times that articles published in the journal in 2006 and 2007 were cited in indexed journals (that is journals indexed in the Thomson Reuters Journal Citation Reports) during 2008.

B = The total number of 'citable items' (usually articles, reviews, proceedings and not editorials or letters) published by that journal in 2006 and 2007.

A/B = 2008 IF

Table 11.2 provides some examples of journal IFs for 2013 (www.impactfactor. weebly.com). For the disciplines of nursing and midwifery IFs of around 2–2.5 would be considered high.

Table 11.2   Journal Impact Factors

Journal	IF 2013
New England Journal of Medicine	51.658
British Journal of Medicine	17.215
Cochrane Database of Systematic Reviews	5.703
Birth: Issues in Perinatal Care	2.926
International Journal of Nursing Studies	2.31
Cancer Nursing	1.878
Midwifery	1.79
Journal of Advanced Nursing	1.65

Source: www.impactfactor.weebly.com

The Importance of Dissemination

There are many reasons for disseminating research findings and each one should be considered equally as important as the next. Ethically, researchers have a responsibility to research participants and to healthcare provision to disseminate any findings from research studies. Of course, this makes sense, as it would be entirely unfair to ask individuals to participate in research and not report the results of the study. This ethical onus on researchers is clearly stated in the Declaration of Helsinki (1964) and it is essential that researchers adhere to this:

... authors have a duty to make publicly available the results of their research on human subjects and are accountable for the completeness and accuracy of their reports ... negative and inconclusive as well as positive results should be published or otherwise made publicly available.

Research must also be reported in an effort to advance healthcare knowledge and scholarship. Consider, for example, other modules that you may be undertaking as part of your course. It is highly likely that you will find research-based evidence informing the content of these modules. In this sense, dissemination of research findings for academics and educationalists is very important so that course content and curriculum development can be informed and up-to-date. Furthermore, in using the findings from high quality research, healthcare practice may be improved. This, however, can only occur when findings are disseminated widely so that they are made accessible to the public, healthcare practitioners and those responsible for policy and guideline development. A prime example of this is the use of research findings and evidence by the National Institute for Health and Care Excellence (www.nice.org.uk) in the UK for developing national guidelines to direct clinical care.

Dissemination of research findings is important also for challenging current clinical practice. On clinical placements you may have heard it said that *'this is the way we have always done it here'* or something similar. Simply doing something because it has always been done that way is not to say that this is the correct or optimum way of doing it. By disseminating findings from research, traditional practices can be evaluated to determine if they reflect contemporary evidence or whether that are outdated and need to change. In this sense, tradition can be challenged and progressed so that optimum healthcare provision, based on sound, high-quality research findings, can be achieved.

A further important reason for disseminating research findings is to facilitate and promote the critique and replication of studies. In most instances, it is recommended that healthcare practice should not be changed on the basis of one research study alone. This is because there is a potential for the findings of single study to result from chance alone. Replication of studies is recommended so that consistencies or inconsistencies in findings can be determined. This will ensure high level, robust evidence and will assist with determining appropriate implementation of research findings. Replication also allows for limitations of previous studies to be addressed and overcome, so that any replicated study may be improved in design and conduct, as necessary.

Research findings, whether positive or negative, have implications for research practice. Additionally, and importantly, research findings have implications for future research. While preliminary research studies might be conducted to inform the development of larger studies (for example, an audit of an outcome or practice may be conducted to determine the sample size for a randomised controlled trial), it is often in the course of research that further questions emerge which warrant investigation. In this sense, research findings can lead to further research study. Consider for example a study that explores the national practices of General Practitioners in prescribing antibiotics. You might expect that practices would be similar across regions and you simply wish to know what these practices are. The study, however, in determining practices also reveals these to be geographically diverse. This in itself provides a surprising finding that now warrants further exploration and a new research question 'Why do practices differ?' emerges. To answer this question, a new study, using a different design, would need to be developed. This is just one example of how research findings in one study can have implications for future research studies.

ACTIVITY 11.2

As an activity, source a paper describing a research study on a topic of interest to you (you could use the paper from Activity 11.1). Read the findings of this study and note down your thoughts on these as follows: i) implications for clinical practice; and ii) implications for future research. From these determine whether any new research questions emerge from the findings. Describe these questions and the type of study design that is needed to answer them. This will help you begin to think about how research can lead to further research and challenge you in determining the most appropriate study design for answering new research questions.

Implementing Findings – Barriers and Facilitators

The process of implementing and using research findings in clinical practice has long been debated and is certainly not without its challenges. By now you are likely to have come across the term 'theory-practice gap', and it is this that healthcare researchers and practitioners are continuously endeavouring to overcome. The theory-practice gap (sometime referred to as the research-practice gap) describes the discrepancy between what emerging new theory or research says we should be doing compared to what we actually are doing in practice. Squires et al. (2011) describe a possible 10-year time lag between research findings and utilisation of these in practice. As alluded to in Chapter 1 of this book, this is not to say that practitioners are unwilling or reluctant to use research findings, rather there are existing barriers, perceived or otherwise, that appear to impede effective research implementation. Some of these barriers include access to research findings, time to read research reports, ability to appraise and utilise research findings, lack of authority to instigate practice change, limited organisational/cultural commitment to change and lack of funding to facilitate change (Glacken & Chaney, 2004; Hutchinson & Johnston, 2004; Squires et al., 2011).

Implementing research findings into practice unquestionably requires a commitment by all involved. Strategies to facilitate effective research implementation remain underdeveloped and are urgently required. Movements in the right direction, however, are taking place. The use of rapid and wide dissemination strategies, for example, should assist with this. Shifts in organisational structures are also helping. For example, an increasing use of practice development coordinators and clinical skills facilitators will help in identifying areas that need change and in ensuring change happens. Mandatory study days for updating clinical skills and knowledge, in-house mini skills workshops and clinical staff participating in research studies are also helping facilitate research implementation. A new and emerging science called 'Implementation Science', which studies methods to promote the integration of research findings and evidence into healthcare policy and practice (Madon et al., 2007) also appears promising for reducing the theory-practice gap. Furthermore, many funding bodies and healthcare organisations now require researchers to document an implementation strategy as part of the development of their study proposal/protocol. Collectively, these endeavours, it is hoped, will assist and increase research implementation in clinical care.

Chapter Summary

The focus of this chapter was to outline for you the importance of research dissemination and implementation. On reading this chapter you should understand that the findings from research studies can significantly impact on what we do and how we do it in clinical practice. It is for this reason that accurate, honest and credible dissemination of research is essential. Numerous strategies may be employed by researchers to disseminate research results. While the list provided in this chapter is not exhaustive, it provides you with the main strategies utilised in healthcare disciplines. It is important also that you understand the merits and limitations of the differing strategies so that you can determine whether a chosen strategy is the most appropriate one for disseminating the findings to the primary target audience. Furthermore, while a more in-depth description on journal publications as a strategy for disseminating research findings was provided, this is not to suggest that this strategy is any more important that other strategies. Rather, as you are most likely to use journals as sources of information during the course of your study, it would be useful for you to have a deeper understanding of this strategy. The importance of disseminating research findings cannot be underestimated and the reasons are multiple. You should now have an understanding of these reasons and their meaning for advancing clinical care, scholarship, knowledge, and future practice. As with many areas of work and indeed life, challenges exist. Implementing research findings is no different. As students of healthcare and future practitioners, the onus is on all of you, individually and collectively, to facilitate research dissemination and evidence-based practice as best as you possibly can.

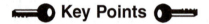

Key Points

- The research process is not complete until the findings of a study have been reported and disseminated.
- In reporting and disseminating research findings, three essential criteria must be met. These are accurate reporting, truthfulness and researcher credibility.
- There are numerous and varied strategies for disseminating research findings. These include healthcare journals, books, theses, conferences, seminars, posters, brochures, flyers, healthcare websites and other media such as radio, television and newspapers. A researcher, in choosing a strategy, must ensure that it is the most appropriate strategy for effective dissemination to the target audience.
- The importance of disseminating research findings cannot be underestimated. Dissemination is important for ethical reasons, for advancing healthcare knowledge and scholarship, for advancing healthcare practice and progress, for challenging tradition, for promoting critique and replication of studies and for identifying new research questions or topics for future study.
- Barriers exist for effective research implementation. It is important that these barriers are overcome. Effective facilitators for implementing research findings should be identified and utilised so that optimum healthcare provision can be attained.

Useful Online Resources

http://impactfactor.weebly.com
www.thelancet.com
www.mdlinx.com/nursing/journals.cfm
www.implementationscience.com/

12

Critically Evaluating Research Studies

Introduction

While research impacted on nursing and the medical professions in the past, since the 1980s there have been attempts to make research more applicable to professional practice. Initially, the approach was an attempt to support practice by reference to research, a concept known as research utilisation (Polit & Beck, 2014). In the 1990s, the idea developed that research should inform practice rather than simply support it and the concept of evidence-based practice was born (Grove et al., 2013). While some support for evidence-based practice came from Systematic Review repositories such as the Cochrane Collaboration, the Centre for Reviews and Dissemination, the National Institute for Clinical Excellence (NICE) and the Scottish Intercollegiate Guidelines Network (SIGN), the advent of research utilisation and evidence-based practice reinforced the need for nurses and other healthcare professionals to be research aware and more adept at critically reading research.

☑ Learning Outcomes ☑

By the end of this chapter you should be able to:

- State why research studies should be read critically
- Critically appraise a piece of research
- Recognise the importance of replication studies in developing strong evidence for practice.

Quality and Integrity of Research

If research is to become the foundation of practice, it is important that the research that is used is of an acceptable standard. The study should be robust and have as few limitations as possible. The nature of limitations in research studies are such that they can vary from being quite minor, to undermining the methodological integrity of the study. While no study is free of limitations it is important to be able to differentiate between a study that is essentially good and one that is fundamentally flawed (Grove et al., 2013).

Most commonly limitations to the integrity of a research study are inadvertent, perhaps due to lack of understanding of the research process, or the nature of the study being undertaken. However, in other instances, the problem can be intentional or of a nature that undermines the rights or safety of participants in which case it most likely falls under the heading of scientific misconduct. Habermann et al., (2010) state that the definition of scientific misconduct includes fabrication, falsification and plagiarism of data, as well as other serious deviations from accepted research practice. Gøtzsche (2009) advocates that readers of research should be like detectives, always watchful and aware that things may not always be as they seem. He adds that poor studies are sometimes disguised to appear to be something they are not and the first step in identifying these studies is by considering all research as potentially flawed, no matter what qualifications the author may hold, and reviewing that research critically.

Critically Reading Research

In undertaking a piece of research, the goal of the researcher is to have as few limitations as possible within the study. However, while all research studies have some limitations, it is important that the reader recognises what those limitations are and how they impact on the findings of the research. If research in healthcare is to be truly evidence based, the concept of critical analysis needs to be embraced. Critical analysis, as well as identifying the strengths and limitations of research studies, and identifying studies that are less than robust, can also help to develop the research skills of both the individual undertaking the analysis and of authors by encouraging critical analysis of their own work before publication. Researchers need to be critical of their own work and be able to recognise the limitations of their research and the consequences this may have for the outcomes. Nonetheless, it is important to recognise that critical analysis is not criticism, and is not a personal attack on the author or a belittling of the researcher's ability. It is a non-emotive, objective form of inquiry that is supported by evidence from the literature.

A critique of a research study may be considered as an in-depth critical analysis of that study and is usually done as an academic exercise. Critiquing tools generally consider all the steps in the research process and are a good way for novice reviewers to check the robustness of a study. In a literature review however, due to word limits, only one or two elements of the critique that highlight the strengths or limitations of a study are usually presented and discussed. There are numerous instruments available for critiquing and critically analysing research studies. Some instruments claim suitability for critiquing all types of studies. However, the counter argument is that the paradigms and philosophies of various methodologies are radically different and that separate instruments are required for the various approaches (Lee, 2006; Ryan et al., 2007). Numerous instruments and checklists are also available for critically analysing systematic reviews, for example Critical Appraisal Skills Programme (CASP) (2010) and Scottish Intercollegiate Guidelines Network (SIGN) (2013).

The purpose of critiquing and critically analysing studies as mentioned earlier is to ensure that research studies that influence practice, or that are used to support concepts within a literature review or a research study, have both a quality of evidence that is relevant and a methodological integrity that demonstrates robustness (Johnson & Taylor, 2014). A guide to determining the relevance and critically evaluating a research study can be found in Table 12.1.

Table 12.1   Guidelines for critically evaluating research study

Determine the relevance of the study	Review the title and the abstract of the study
Read the study	Read the study and become familiar with the purpose, the methodology used and identify and appraise the methods used in the steps of the research process
Identify the strengths and limitations	Offer examples and support from the literature
Recommendations for future studies in the field	Identify how the study could be improved
Overall evaluation of the study	This is an indication of how the study is rated in the context of the robustness of the study and its contribution to the topic being studied

Relevance

When undertaking a search of the literature for either clinical or academic reasons, research studies and articles are often identified that are of little or no relevance to the current search. As time constraints are often an issue when undertaking these searches it is important to determine which studies are relevant and which ones are unwanted. Some factors that may be considered when attempting to determine relevance are displayed in Table 12.2.

Table 12.2   Factors influencing relevance

Title	The report title should identify what the study is about in a clear and unambiguous way. This is often the first indicator that a study may be relevant
Abstract	This should offer a clear overview of the study, identifying the key steps in the research process including the purpose, methodology, main findings and recommendations. It should be clearer now if this study is relevant to your needs
Author	The professional experiences and /or qualifications of the author suggest a knowledge or expertise in this particular field of enquiry. This may be particularly relevant if the author is well known for research in this area

The initial exposure to any research study is usually through the title and/or the abstract. This is often the first indicator of the focus, and thus the relevance, of the study to the reader. The title should clearly identify the purpose of the study, so the reader is left in no doubt as to what the study is about. If examining studies in relation to a clinical or research problem, this is often where studies are excluded. If the title appears relevant then the next step is to review the abstract.

The abstract should briefly discuss the purpose, methodology, main findings, conclusions and recommendations of the study. At this stage, the reader should be able to determine if the focus of the study corresponds with, and is relevant to, the research or clinical problem being investigated (Rebar et al., 2011). Another factor that can help to determine how relevant the study can be is the author's qualifications and/or professional experience. This is particularly the case where the study appears to fit the criteria being sought, and the researcher is known to have an expertise in this area.

Identifying the Steps in the Research Process

After determining the relevance of the study the next step is to read the study carefully and identify the steps in the research process and how meticulously they were followed. There are methodological differences in the research steps between various research methodologies. Therefore, when evaluating the robustness of a study, it is important that the reviewer has a good understanding of the steps in the research process and also a good understanding of the methodology being employed in the article being reviewed. For example, in quantitatively-based research the purpose of the literature review is to study the available literature, refine the research problem and it may also influence the methodological approach adopted to the study. To do this it needs to be undertaken early in the research study. In qualitatively-based research the purpose of a literature review is to gather information in relation to available knowledge on the phenomenon of interest and to support the themes that arise from the study. In some qualitative approaches such as Grounded Theory and Phenomenology the main review of the literature may be undertaken after the data is gathered to reduce the risk of the researcher being prejudiced by previous studies (Coughlan et al., 2013). An overview of the steps in the process has been included in Table 12.3 and instruments for reviewing quantitative and qualitative studies and systematic reviews can be found on the website for this book.

Table 12.3   Steps in the Research Process

Steps in the research process	
Logical Consistency	Is the study presented in a logical order following the steps of the research?
Purpose	Was the research problem / significance of the study clearly identified?
Review of the Literature	Was a review of the literature undertaken?
Research Question/ Hypothesis	Has a research question / hypothesis been identified?
Methodology/Philosophical underpinning	Has the research methodology/philosophical underpinnings been discussed?

Steps in the research process

Data Gathering Method	Has the method of collecting data been described? Is it appropriate for this study?
Validity/Reliability/ Rigour	Was the robustness of the data-gathering instrument/data ensured?
Sample	Was the method by which the sample was selected discussed? Was the target population described? Was the selection method appropriate for the approach used?
Ethical Considerations	Were all the ethical principles considered and adhered to? Was ethical approval granted for this study?
Data Analysis	Was data analysis discussed? Was it appropriate for the study?
Findings	Were the findings appropriately presented?
Discussion	Were the findings discussed with reference to the literature review? Did the author discuss the strengths and limitations of the study?
Conclusions/Implications/ Recommendations	Will the findings of this study be of interest to the profession? Were the implications for clinical practice identified? Were recommendations made as to how future research might develop the findings of this study?
References	Were all the texts, journal articles, websites and other media sources referred to in the study accurately referenced?

Identifying the Strengths and Limitations

Critically appraising a research study is not simply a case of identifying how well the steps were adhered to, but also recognising what the implications of a strength or limitation might be. Examples of the strengths and limitations should be presented along with supporting evidence from a textbook or article. It is always crucial to remember that a critical analysis is objective and not a personal opinion. Therefore, analysis must always be supported by evidence. A critical appraisal of a sample of a research study can be seen in the box below.

Critical Appraisal of a Research Study

Young Singaporean women's knowledge of cervical cancer and pap smear screening: a descriptive study (Shea et al., 2013: 3312–3)

A cross-sectional descriptive correlational design was used to assess the knowledge of pap smear and cervical cancer of young Singaporean females and their intention towards future uptake of pap smears.

(Continued)

(Continued)

Sample and Setting

Convenience sampling was used to recruit Singaporean women aged 18–25 at a university with a full-time female undergraduate population of 13,066 as of year 2011 (National Registry of Diseases Office of Singapore, 2011). The convenience sampling method was best suited for this study as the minimally required sample size was large, and it was a fast, inexpensive and easy-to-use method, especially when potential subjects are readily accessible (Polgar & Thomas, 2008).

Data Collection

Female students were approached by one of the researchers during recreational time around campus at various sites such as canteens and lecture halls. Eligible participants were invited to participate in the research study, and the purpose of the study was explained to them. 460 questionnaires were distributed and 426 (92.61 per cent) of them were returned. However, only 393 questionnaires were accepted as some of those who completed the questionnaire did not fit the selection criteria (e.g. outside of age range, non-Singaporean). The questionnaires were self-administered by the participants.

Source: Shea et al. (2013: 3312–3)

Critical Analysis

In Shea et al.'s (2013) study, the researchers opted to use convenience sampling in one university campus. Polit and Beck (2014) state that convenience samples, which choose individuals as they are readily available, fall into the category of non-probability sampling, and that as such this sample is more likely to be atypical and therefore less likely to be representative of the population. Also the researchers selected their sample from one site. Grove et al. (2013) state that homogeneity can have the effect of limiting the results to the subjects in the study. Thus overall the findings of this study should be read with caution if attempting to generalise the results.

While no study is without limitations, it is important that researchers can recognise and identify limitations within their own work. In Shea et al.'s (2013) study the authors recognise the limitation associated with using convenience sampling and other issues in their study (see the box below). Recognition of limitations by the author of a study increases the reader's confidence in the trustworthiness and robustness of the research. Therefore when critically appraising a study, if the authors have identified a limitation that is being reported this should be acknowledged.

Limitations of a Study as Identified by the Authors

Young Singaporean women's knowledge of cervical cancer and pap smear screening: a descriptive study

Limitations of Study

The study used a cross-sectional design, thus is limited in its ability to draw a causal relationship between the variables across time. However, the data collected can still provide knowledge on concurrent relationship between the variables tested and the study population (Parahoo, 2006; Polit & Beck, 2010). The results from the study may not be generalisable to all Singaporean young women as the participants were recruited from only one university (Parahoo, 2006). Therefore, results need to be interpreted with caution. Convenience sampling was used in this study, and thus, the study is subject to inherent bias (investigator/sampling bias) which might cause the results to be unrepresentative of the population being studied (Polit & Beck, 2010). As the questionnaires were self-reported by the participants, the study might also be subject to self-reporting bias (or response set bias) in the data obtained (Polit & Beck, 2010).

Source: Shea et al. (2013: 3316–7)

Recommendations for Future Studies

Having reviewed a study and identified its strengths and weaknesses, the next step is to recommend how these strengths might be enhanced and the limitations overcome. There is also an opportunity to identify gaps that appear in the study. Both these offer an opportunity to the reviewer, especially if this analysis is being performed as part of a research study, as the limitations of previous studies can be avoided and the identified gaps may form an important part of the study being undertaken.

Overall Evaluation of the Study

Having critically analysed the study, identified its strengths and limitations and how these impact on the outcomes of the research, and finally made recommendations that would strengthen future studies, the next step is to make an overall evaluation of the study. This is about establishing the trustworthiness and significance of the work. This includes determining if the methodology chosen was suited to the research problem or hypothesis, how faithful the researcher was to the chosen methodology and how precisely the steps of the research process were integrated into the methodology. It can be helpful at this stage to compare and contrast the outcomes of this study with others to see if there is support for the findings. Ultimately, this stage is about determining whether, and to what degree, the outcomes of this study impact on nursing knowledge and practice.

Replication of Research

Another way of testing the accuracy of a study's findings is through the replication of that research study (Polit & Beck, 2014). Replication studies include exact replication, which is a repeat of the original study; approximate replication where the methodology of the original study is replicated; and systematic replication which is undertaken using a different methodology and approach to investigate the same phenomenon. All are performed to verify the outcomes of the original study (Grove et al., 2013). Replication studies have an important role in the development of robust evidence for practice. Despite this, these types of studies are often wrongly regarded as less scholarly, with preference being given to original research. Nonetheless, it is important to remember, that evidence-based practice refers to the evidence of multiple studies and not simply one piece of research. It is thus important to have both replication and original studies to ensure both the quality and integrity of the research underpinning best practice.

Chapter Summary

Healthcare professions in the twenty-first century are rapidly becoming governed by the principle that best practice is guided by robust research evidence. In order for nurses and other healthcare professionals to engage fully in practice that is evidence based they need to become more research aware and more adept at critically reading research. Research that is going to underpin practice cannot simply be accepted at face value. It must be questioned and tested on an ongoing basis in the light of new developments and new research. If healthcare professionals are to offer the best care to their patients and clients they need to continually update their knowledge of the research that underpins their practice.

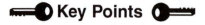
Key Points

- Research should never be taken at face value.
- When reading research it should be read critically.
- Replication studies are an important way of testing outcomes of previous studies.

Glossary

Accessible population (Study population)   This is a portion of the target population that a researcher can easily access. The accessible population needs to be representative of the target population if inferences to the target population are to be made.

Action research   Action research incorporates working with participants in a specific situation to problem solve an issue that is identified as needing development/improvement and identification and enactment of an intervention (change) to achieved the desired outcome.

Apriori coding   A template of possible codes is created before the formal analysis process begins.

Autonomy   Respect for a person's right to self-determination and freedom of choice.

Beneficence   Doing good.

Bivariate analysis   The comparison of two variables to determine if there is a relationship between them.

Categorical data   Data such as nominal and ordinal level that can be categorised into distinct groups but have no inherent numerical value.

Case study   Case study is the study of single or multiple cases (unit, group or entity) in its own right. The cases have clear boundaries and are studied in context because they always occur in a physical and social setting.

Causal-comparative/ex-post-facto designs   Non-experimental designs that are closest to an experiment because the research question is causal but it is not possible to manipulate the independent variable.

Causal relationship   A relationship whereby a change in one variable causes a change in another variable.

Census   This is a study where data is gathered from the entire target population.

Central tendency   The single value that represents the distribution of the data. There are three measures of central tendency namely the mode, the median and the mean.

Clinical equipoise   A state of uncertainty about the benefits of treatments being evaluated in a randomised clinical trial.

Coercion   Forcing or placing undue pressure or influence on a person.

Commissioned study   A study in which an external funding body, such as a professional organisation, a government department or a private funding source, has requested that research on a particular topic be done.

Competence   Having the ability or necessary skills to perform an action.

Concept analysis   This is a review of the literature to determine the attributes and characteristics of a concept.

Continuous data   Data that have a numerical value such as interval and ratio level and can be measured along a continuum.

Correlation co-efficient (r)   Is a number between −1.0 (perfect negative correlation) and 1.0 (perfect positive correlation) that represents the strength of the relationship between two or more variables. 0.0 indicates no relationship. A positive correlation means the variables move in the same direction while a negative correlation means they move in opposite directions.

Correlational designs   Non-experimental designs that can measure or test the relationship between two or more variables.

Correlation indices   A calculation of the existence and/or strength of a relationship between two variables.

Credibility   Accuracy and truth in research findings.

Critical analysis   An appraisal of the quality of a research study. Unlike a critique in that only significant strengths / limitations of the study are presented.

Critical/transformative/participatory/advocacy paradigm   Paradigms that are concerned with social conditions and a critique of the known structure of society. Advocacy and participatory world views draw on critical theory and their focus is on enablement, empowerment and emancipation.

Critique   A critical examination of a research study that identifies the strengths and limitations of that study. It is often undertaken as an academic exercise.

Data saturation   This is said to be achieved when no new themes are emerging from the data and participants' descriptions reflect previous data gathered. It is an indicator that data collection can cease.

Deduction   Commonly referred to as 'general to specific'. In research, testing of an existing theory takes place and is then either accepted, rejected or modified. Associated with theory testing research.

Deontology   An ethical theory which focuses on duty and obligation in research.

Descriptive/observational designs   Non-experimental designs that broadly focus on observing or describing a phenomenon to provide a precise account of its existence or nature, its prevalence and/or distribution.

Descriptive statistics   Analysis that is undertaken to describe the characteristics of those involved in a study. The most common features that involve analysis of one variable at a time (univariate analysis) are frequency/distribution, central tendency and dispersion/measures of variability.

Dispersion/measures of variability   Measures of dispersion offer insight into the spread (dispersion) of scores in a set of data.

Dissemination   The spreading, circulation or dispersal of something, especially information, widely.

Documentary sources   Any form of records related to the lives of individuals, groups, communities or societies.

Frequency distribution   Concerned with how many times a value appears in the data. These can be presented as actual numbers (n), percentages or category (where there are large numbers).

Epistemology   The branch of philosophy that studies the history of knowledge.

Empiricism   The opposite of rationalism, empiricism is located in the belief that our knowledge is derived from our experiences of the world. The vehicles for our experiences are our senses.

Ethics   A branch of moral philosophy concerned with that which is right or wrong, good or bad, fair or unfair.

Ethnography   Ethnography is the study of the culture and social structure of groups and has its roots in anthropology.

Exclusion criteria   These are conditions whose presence or absence, depending on the study, will exclude individuals from the target population.

Experimental designs   Concerned with conducting experiments and include three elements: intervention, control and randomisation.

Gatekeeper   A person, organisation, group or platform that allows or denies people access to participating in a research study.

Generalisability   The ability to extend or apply a study's findings to individuals outside of the study sample in the wider, general community.

Grounded theory   In grounded theory methodology a systematic set of procedures are used to develop theory that is 'grounded' in the data.

Guttman Scale   A cumulative scale where respondents tick statements with which they agree. It is hierarchical, that is, when a person ticks a statement with which they agree it is likely that they will also agree with statements lower down in the hierarchy.

Heterogeneity   Diversity or differences in some element, for example practices or populations.

Homogeneity   The opposite of heterogeneity and refers to similarity in elements.

Hypothesis   A statement that expresses a relationship between two or more variables that will be examined in a study. It may be considered a prediction of the possible results of a study.

Inclusion criteria   These are distinct conditions that will identify those who will be included in the target population.

Induction   Commonly referred to as 'specific to general'. In research, it is where enough observations and measurements of a phenomenon are made until a confident generalisation can be made. Associated with theory generating research.

Inductive coding   Coding directly from the data in analysis of narrative (words).

Integrative review   This is an all-encompassing review of the literature (experimental, non-experimental, theoretical and conceptual) whose aim is to offer an in-depth understanding of a phenomenon.

Inferential statistics   Analysis that attempts to establish if there is a relationship between variables; making inferences (predictions) about the wider population from which the sample was drawn and assessing the probability that the outcomes of the study are dependable and did not happen by chance.

Interpretivism/Constructivism   Paradigms whose central belief is that reality is constructed through the meanings human beings develop as a result of their experiences and their interactions with others in a social world.

Interview   A formal dialogue between two or more people for the purpose of eliciting information about a phenomenon of interest. Can be undertaken in person, on the telephone or through electronic media.

Journal impact factor   A measure that reflects the frequency with which a journal's articles are cited in the scientific literature. It is often used as a proxy measure for the relative importance of a journal within its field.

Justice   Fairness and equity.

Levels of data   Refers to the type of numerical data collected in a research study. There are four main types, that is, nominal, ordinal, interval and ratio.

Level of significance   This refers to the degree to which a finding probably occurred by chance. This is usually set at less than or equal to 0.05 per cent; meaning that chance will only play a role in this finding at worst five times in every 100.

Lexical semantics   The analysis of word meanings and relations between them.

Likert Scale   A scale that measures level of agreement with a series of pre-defined statements.

Measurement Scale   A series of questions that measures or tests variables related to a phenomenon.

Meta-analysis   A statistical pooling of results from all of the individual studies reporting on an identified outcome in order to provide an overall single result for that outcome.

Methodological   Pertaining to a body of strict practices and procedures or a set of working methods used by those engaging in a process of inquiry.

Mixed method   Mixed method studies that combine or blend methods that are normally associated with different paradigms in one study.

Multivariate analysis   The comparison of more than two variables to see if there is a relationship between them.

Narrative review   Also known as a traditional literature review. It should be undertaken in a systematic manner, with clear review strategies and searches that are systematic in nature.

Narrative research   Narrative research refers to spoken or written text that gives an account of something (event(s) and/or action(s)) that are connected.

Non-experimental design   All studies that are not experimental or quasi-experimental.

Non-maleficence   Avoidance of harm.

Non-probability sample   This is a sample that is probably not representative of the target population. Convenience and purposive samples are examples.

Non-response bias   A potentially inaccurate presumption that can be made by not accounting for the non-responders in a survey.

Normal distribution   Demonstrates the spread of the scores in a data set. Data that are normally distributed produce a 'bell' shape when scores are plotted on a graph. Also known as a 'Gaussian' curve. In a bell curve most data are concentrated around the centre with the frequency of scores falling off at either side.

Null hypothesis (Statistical hypothesis)   This is a testable statement asserting that there is no relationship between two or more variables. By statistically rejecting the null-hypothesis the researcher accepts the hypothesis as true.

Observation   Where a researcher directly observes phenomena in the natural setting or context.

Paradigm   Definitions vary but all refer to a 'pattern', 'example' or 'exemplar'. Most quoted definition is that of Kuhn (1970) who describes a paradigm as the underlying assumptions and intellectual structures that direct research and development in a given field.

Personal knowledge   Knowledge by 'acquaintance'. Associated with having experience of something.

Phenomenon   A phenomenon is an aspect of reality that can be experienced or sensed. Phenomena when labelled are known as concepts.

Phenomenology   Phenomenology is a philosophy rather than a scientific method that underpins a variety of methods for studying and understanding individuals' 'lived experiences'.

Placebo   A dummy treatment, for example, a sugar pill.

Population   May be defined as all the components that are deemed to have one or more common characteristics and therefore constitute a group.

Positivism/post-positivism   Paradigms that underpin the scientific method with prediction, generalisation, measurement, observables and researcher objectivity as key features.

Power analysis   A statistical test to identify the sample size required to prevent a Type II sampling error.

Probability   The likelihood that the results were not obtained by chance alone if the null hypothesis is true. Assuming that the null hypothesis is true the p value tells researchers how rarely they would observe a difference as large (or larger) than the one they did.

Probability sample   This is a sample that is probably representative of the target population. Simple random and stratified random samples are examples.

Procedural knowledge   Knowledge 'how'. Associated with the practical knowledge of how to do something.

Propositional knowledge   Knowledge 'that'. Associated with theories, facts, laws.

Prospective correlation study   A study that recruits participants and follows them forward in time to determine any relationships between the variables under examination in the study.

Qualitative descriptive/Exploratory design   Research methodology whose purpose is to describe/explore a phenomenon/problem/issue. Can encompass a broad range of questions relating to people's experiences, knowledge, attitudes, feelings, perceptions and/or views.

Quasi-experiment   Similar to an experiment in that the manipulation of an intervention is always present but the criteria of control and randomisation may be missing.

Questionnaire   A document that contains a series of questions designed to obtain information about a phenomenon of interest. Can incorporate tests or scales.

Randomised controlled trial   A study, in which participants are allocated to two, or more, groups by random (i.e. by chance). The participants in each group receive a different treatment.

Rationalism   Located in the belief that propositional knowledge comes to us through the use of reason.

Reliability   Consistency in measurement instruments and dependable study results.

Representativeness   This is the degree to which a sample reflects the characteristics of the population from which it was drawn; thus the term representative sample.

Research question   This is a clearly defined question that a researcher intends to seek an answer to, in the course of a research study.

Rigour   Extreme thoroughness and accuracy in research achieved through strict methods, processes or procedures.

Sample   A selection of individuals or items used to illustrate the possible responses or behaviours of the population.

Sample frame   All of the individuals who are part of the total population.

Sampling bias   Inaccuracy in sampling that leads to an over representation of one or more subgroups within the sample.

Scoping review   A scoping review also known as a scoping project/scoping study is a review undertaken to identify the scope or range of literature that is available on a particular topic or broad research question.

Sensitive data   Data related to private issues or issues which people find embarrassing, threatening or emotionally difficult to discuss.

Significance level   The level at which the researcher is prepared to accept or reject the null hypothesis. It is commonly set at 1/20 or 0.05 and expressed as a probability value, for example, $p \leq 0.05$. In certain situations a smaller p value may be set, for instance, $p \leq 0.01$.

Standard deviation   A measure that calculates the dispersion of the scores in a dataset in relation to the mean.

Surveys   Surveys are a widely used data collection method in the application of non-experimental research that gathers numerical data.

Systematic review   A method of enquiry that brings together all of the studies on a particular topic in one place to answer a specific review question.

Target population (Theoretical population)   All individuals or units that are deemed by the researcher to have one or more common characteristics and from whom the sample will be drawn.

Theory   Theory provides knowledge about the world in which we live through research. There are multiple, conflicting definitions of theory but there are some common characteristics:

- Theory is concerned with some aspect of the world.
- Speculates on how reality might be or ought to be.
- Theories are never certain and always subject to change.
- Theories are comprised of phenomena (concepts).
- Theories are comprised of propositions that identify the nature of the relationship between concepts.

Theory generating research   Research that generates theories usually inductively.

Theory-practice gap   The discrepancy between theoretical/scientific knowledge and how care is given in clinical practice.

Theory testing/validating research   Research that tests/validates theories usually deductively.

Trustworthiness   Trust in the findings of a study and knowing them to be reliable and true.

Type II sampling error   Occurs when, as a result of a sample size that is too small, there is a failure to reject the null hypothesis and demonstrate significance in a statistical test.

Univariate analysis   The analysis of one variable for the purpose of describing it.

Utilitarianism   An ethical theory that supports research where the greatest benefit for the greatest number of people is central.

Validity   Accuracy, truth and soundness in study design and conduct.

Virtue ethics   An ethical theory that is concerned with how a researcher behaves and the quality of his/her character in making decisions and judgments.

References

Anderson, S., Allen, P., Peckham, S., Goodwin, N. (2008) Asking the right questions: scoping studies in the commissioning of research on the organisation and delivery of health services. *Health Research and Policy Systems*. (6)7. Available at: www.ncbi.nlm.nih.gov/pmc/articles/PMC2500008/pdf/1478-4505-6-7.pdf (accessed 15 November 2013).

Andrews, T. (2012) What is social constructionism? *Grounded Theory Review*. 11(1). Available at: http://groundedtheoryreview.com/2012/06/01/what-is-social-constructionism/ (accessed 20 November 2013).

Annells, M. (2007) Guest editorial: What's common with qualitative research these days? *Journal of Clinical Nursing*. 16(2): 223–4.

Arksey, H., O'Malley, L. (2005) Scoping studies: towards a methodological framework. *International Journal of Social Research Methodology*. 8(1): 19–32.

Asaria, P., MacMahon, E. (2006) Measles in the United Kingdom: can we eradicate it by 2010? *British Medical Journal*. 333(7474): 890–95.

Aveyard, H. (2010) *Doing a Literature Review in Health and Social Care*, 2nd edn. Maidenhead: Open University Press.

Bath, B.M.W., Watson, A.R. (2009) Need for ethics approval and patient consent in clinical research. *Stroke*. 40: 1555–6.

Baumbusch, J.L. (2011) Conducting critical ethnography in long-term residential care: experiences of a novice researcher in the field. *Journal of Advanced Nursing*. 67(1): 184–92.

Bazeley, P. (2013) *Qualitative Data Analysis: Practical Strategies*. Los Angeles: Sage.

BBC News. (2001) Organ scandal background. Available at: http://news.bbc.co.uk/2/hi/1136723.stmm (accessed 30 June 2013).

Beauchamp, T.L., Childress J.F. (2013) *Principles of Biomedical Ethics*, 7th edn. NewYork: Oxford University Press.

Benton, D.C., Cormack, D.F.S. (2000) *The Research Process in Nursing*, 4th edn. Oxford: Blackwell Science.

Bettany-Saltikov, J. (2012) *How To Do a Systematic Literature Review in Nursing: A Step-by-Step Guide*. Maidenhead: Open University Press.

Bettany-Saltikov, J., Whittaker, V.J. (2013) Selecting the most appropriate inferential statistical test for your quantitative research study. *Journal of Clinical Nursing*. 22(15–16): 2244–52.

Bircumshaw, D. (1990) The utilization of research findings in clinical nursing practice. *Journal of Advanced Nursing*. 15: 1272–80.

Bland, M., Altman, D.G. (1997) Statistics notes: Cronbach's alpha. *British Medical Journal*. 314: 512.

Botti, M., Endacott, R. (2008) Clinical research 5: quantitative data collection and analysis. *International Emergency Nursing*. 16: 132–7.

Brett Davis, M. (2007) *Doing a Successful Research Project*. Houndmills: Palgrave Macmillan.

Brown, C.E., Ecoff, L., Kim, S.C., Wickline, M.A., Rose, B., Klimpel, K., Glaser, D. (2010) Multi-institutional study of barriers to research utilisation and evidence-based practice among hospital nurses. *Journal of Clinical Nursing*. 19: 1944–51.

Burns, N., Grove, S. (2005) *The Practice of Nursing Research: Conduct, Critique and Utilization*, 5th edn. Philadelphia: Elsevier.

Centre for Disease Control and Prevention. (2011) *US Public Health Service Syphilis Study at Tuskegee*. Available at: www.cdc.gov/tuskegee/clintonp.htm (accessed 13 August 2013).

Chen, S.H., Shao, J.H., Hsiao, Y.C., Lee, H.C. (2013) Barriers to research utilization by registered nurses in Taiwan. *Research in Nursing and Health.* 36: 191–202.

Chien, W. (2010) A survey of nurses' perceived barriers to research utilisation in Hong Kong. *Journal of Clinical Nursing.* 19: 3584–6.

Christie, J., Hamill, C., Power, J. (2012) How can we maximize nursing students' learning about research evidence and utilization in undergraduate, preregistration programmes? A discussion paper. *Journal of Advanced Nursing.* 68(12): 2789–2801.

Clandinin, J.D., Connelly, F.M. (2000) *Narrative Inquiry: Experience and Story in Qualitative Research.* San Francisco: Jossey-Bass.

Clarke, M. (2006) Systematic review and meta-analysis of quantitative research: overview of methods (part 1, chapter 1). In: Webb, C., Roe, B. (eds), *Reviewing Research Evidence for Nursing Practice: Systematic.* Oxford: Blackwell Publishing.

Clout, L., (2007) Forget the doctor, says TV Gillian McKeith. *The Telegraph,* 13 February. Available at: www.telegraph.co.uk/news/uknews/1542500/Forget-the-doctor-says-TV-Gillian-McKeith.html (accessed 22 April 2014).

Cobban, S.J., Profetto-McGrath, J. (2011) Dental hygienists' research utilization: influence of context and attitudes. *International Journal of Dental Hygiene.* 9: 191–8.

Coenen, M., Basedow-Rajwich, B., König, N., Kesselring, J., Cieza, A. (2011) Functioning and disability in multiple sclerosis from the patient perspective. *Chronic Illness.* 7(4): 291–310.

Colaizzi, P.F. (1978) Pyschological research as a phenomenologist views it. In Valle, R.S., King, M. (eds), *Existential-phenomenological Alternatives for Psychology.* New York: Oxford University Press. pp. 48–71.

Columbia University. (2011) *The Cloning Scandal of Hwang Woo-Suk.* Available at: www.stemcellbioethics.wikischolars.columbia.edu/The+Cloning+Scandal+of+Hwang+Woo-Suk (accessed 7 September 2013).

Comfort, N. (2009) The prisoner as a model organism: malaria research at Stateville Penitentiary. *Studies in the History and Philosophy of Biological and Biomedical Sciences.* 40: 190–203.

Conjoint Faculties Research Ethics Board. (2000) *Instructions for Ethics Review Applicants.* Belfast: Queens University.

Cook, C. (2012) Email interviewing: generating data with a vulnerable population. *Journal of Advanced Nursing.* 68(6): 1330–39.

Cooke, A., Mills, T.A., Lavender, T. (2012) Advanced maternal age: delayed childbearing is rarely a conscious choice. A qualitative study of women's views and experiences. *International Journal of Nursing Studies.* 49(1): 30–9.

Coughlan, M., Cronin, P., Ryan, F. (2007) Step-by-step guide to critiquing research. Part 1: quantitative research. *British Journal of Nursing.* 16(11): 658–63.

Coughlan, M., Cronin, P., Ryan, F. (2009) Survey research: process and limitations. *International Journal of Therapy and Rehabilitation.* 16(1): 9–15.

Coughlan, M., Cronin, P., Ryan, F. (2013) *Doing a Literature Review in Nursing, Health and Social Care.* London: Sage.

Creswell, J.W. (2007) *Qualitative Inquiry & Research Design: Choosing Among Five Approaches,* 2nd edn. Thousand Oaks, CA: Sage.

Creswell, J.W. (2009) *Research Design: Qualitative, Quantitative and Mixed Methods Approaches,* 3rd edn. London: Sage.

Critical Appraisal Skills Programme (2010) Appraisal tools. Available at: www.caspinternational.org/?o=1012 (accessed 2 March 2014).

Cronin, P., Begley, C. (2013) Living with chronic pancreatitis: a qualitative study. *Chronic Illness.* 9(3): 233–47.

Cronin, P., Ryan, F., Coughlan, M. (2008) Undertaking a literature review: a step-by-step approach. *British Journal of Nursing.* 17(1): 38–43.

Cronin, P., Ryan, F., Coughlan, M. (2010) Concept analysis in healthcare research. *International Journal of Therapy and Rehabilitation.* 17(2): 62–8.

Crowley, P. (2006) Prophylactic corticosteroids for preterm birth. *Cochrane Database of Systematic Reviews*. Issue 3. Art. No: CD000065.

Crown, (Elizabeth II). (2004) *Human Tissue Act*. London: The Stationery Office.

Czuber-Dochan, W., Dibley, L.B., Terry, H., Ream, E., Norton, C. (2013) The experience of fatigue in people with inflammatory bowel disease: an exploratory study. *Journal of Advanced Nursing*. 69(9): 1987–99.

Daniel, J. (2012) *Sampling Essentials: Practical Guidelines for Making Sampling Choices*. Los Angeles: Sage.

Daya, S. (2004) Clinical equipoise. *Evidence-based Obstetrics & Gynecology*. 6: 1–2.

De Angelis, C., Drazen, J., Frizelle, F. (2004) Clinical trial registration: a statement from the International Committee of Medical Journal Editors. *New England Journal of Medicine*. 351: 1250–1.

Deloitte. (2012) *Deloitte 2012 Survey of US Health Care Consumers: The Performance of the Health Care System and Health Care Reform*. Washington: Deloitte Center for Health Solutions. Available at: www.deloitte.com/centerforhealthsolutions.

Dickerson, K., Davis, B., Dixon, D. (2004) The Society for Clinical Trials supports United States legislation mandating trial registration. *Clinical Trials*. 1: 417–20.

Donabedian, A. (1988) The quality of care: how can it be assessed? *Journal of American Medical Association (JAMA)*. 260(12): 1743–8.

Doran, T.G. (1981) There's a S.M.A.R.T. way to write management's goals and objectives. *Management Review*. 70(11): 35–6.

Dowling M., Cooney A. (2012) Research approaches related to phenomenology: negotiating a complex landscape. *Nurse Researcher*. 20(2): 21–7.

Draucker, C.B., Martsolf, D.S., Ross, R., Rusk, T.B. (2007) Theoretical sampling and category development in Grounded Theory. *Qualitative Health Research*. 17(8): 1137–48.

Dunne, C. (2011) The place of the literature review in grounded theory research. *International Journal of Social Research Methodology*. 14(2): 111–24.

Effective Public Health Practice Project. (2009) *Quality Assessment Tool*. Available at: www.ephpp.ca/Tools.html (accessed 4 April 2014).

Ellis, P. (2010) *Understanding Research for Nursing Students*. Exeter: Learning Matters.

Ely, C., Scott, I. (2007) *Essential Study Skills for Nursing*. Edinburgh: Mosby.

Estabrooks, C.A. (1999a) The conceptual structure of research utilization. *Research in Nursing & Health*. 22: 203–16.

Estabrooks, C.A. (1999b) Modelling the individual determinants of research utilization. *Western Journal of Nursing Research*. 21(6): 758–72.

Fewell, F. (2005) *An Evaluation of How We Determine Competence in Massage, Aromatherapy, Reflexology and Lymphatic Drainage*. London: Institute for Complementary Medicine.

Fleming, V., Gaidys, U., Robb, Y. (2003) Hermeneutic research in nursing: developing a Gadamerian-based research method. *Nursing Inquiry*. 10(2): 113–20.

Forsman, H., Gustavsson, P., Ehrenberg, A., Rudman, A., Wallin, L. (2009) Research use in clinical practice – extent and patterns among nurses one and three years postgraduation. *Journal of Advanced Nursing*. 65(6): 1195–206.

Freeman, J., Walters, S. (2010) Examining relationships in Quantitative Data. In Gerrish, K., Lacey, A. (eds), *The Research Process in Nursing*, 6th edn. Oxford: Wiley-Blackwell. pp. 455–472.

Gardiner, P. (2003) A virtue ethics approach to moral dilemmas in medicine. *Journal of Medical Ethics*. 29: 297–302.

Gerhard, T. (2008) Bias: considerations for research practice. *American Journal of Health-Systems Pharmacy*, 65: 2159–68.

Gerrish, K. (2010) Evidence-based practice. In Gerrish, K., Lacey, A. (eds), *The Research Process in Nursing*, 6th edn. Oxford: Wiley-Blackwell. pp. 488–500.

Gerrish, K., Ashworth, P., Lacey, A., Bailey, J. (2008) Developing evidence-based practice: experiences of senior and junior clinical nurses. *Journal of Advanced Nursing*. 62(1): 62–73.

Gerrish, K., Guillaume, L. (2006) Whither survey research? The challenge of undertaking postal surveys within the UK research governance framework. *Journal of Research in Nursing.* 11(6): 485–97.

Ghersi, D., Pang, T. (2009) From Mexico to Mali: four years in the history of clinical trial registration. *Journal of Evidence-based Medicine.* 2: 1–7.

Glacken, M., Chaney, D. (2004) Perceived barriers and facilitators to implementing research findings in the Irish setting. *Journal of Clinical Nursing*, 13: 731–40.

Giorgi, A. (1997) The theory, practice and evaluation of the phenomenological method as a qualitative research procedure. *Journal of Phenomenological Psychology.* 28(2): 235–61.

Giorgi, A. (2000a) The status of Husserlian phenomenology in caring research. *Scandinavian Journal of Caring Sciences.* 14: 3–10.

Giorgi, A. (2000b) Concerning the application of phenomenology to caring research. *Scandinavian Journal of Caring Sciences.* 14: 11–15.

Giorgi, A. (2006) Concerning variations in the application of the phenomenologic method. *The Humanistic Psychologist.* 34(4): 305–19.

Glaser, B., Strauss, A. (1967) *The Discovery of Grounded Theory: Strategies for Qualitative Research.* New York: Aldine De Gruyter.

Godlee, F., Smith, J., Marcovitch, H. (2011) Wakefield's article linking MMR vaccine and autism was fraudulent. *British Medical Journal.* 342: c7452.

Golafshani, N. (2003). Understanding reliability and validity in qualitative research. *The Qualitative Report.* 8(4): 597–607.

Goldacre, B. (2008) *Bad Science.* London: Harper Collins Publishers.

Goldacre, B. (2012) *Bad Pharma: How Drug Companies Mislead Doctors and Harm Patients.* London: Harper Collins Publishers.

Gøtzsche P.C. (2009) Readers as research detectives. *Trials.* Available at: www.trialsjournal. com./content/10/1/2.

Greenhalgh, T., Peacock, R. (2005) Effectiveness and efficiency of search methods in systematic reviews of complex evidence: audit of primary sources. *British Medical Journal.* 331(7524): 1064–5.

Grove, S.K., Burns, N., Gray, J.R. (2013) *The Practice of Nursing Research: Appraisal, Synthesis and Generation of Evidence*, 7th edn. St. Louis: Elsevier.

Guba, E.G. (1981) Criteria for assessing the trustworthiness of naturalistic inquiries. *Educational Communication and Technology Journal.* 29: 75–91.

Gupta, R.K., Best, J. McMahon, E. (2005) Mumps and the UK epidemic. *British Medical Journal.* 330: 1132–35.

Guyatt, G., Cook, D., Haynes, B. (2004) Evidence-based medicine has come a long way. *British Medical Journal.* 329: 390–1.

Habermann, B., Broome M., Pryor, E.R., Ziner, K.W. (2010) Research coordinators' experiences with scientific misconduct and research integrity. *Nursing Research.* 59(1): 51–7.

Hamberg, K., Johansson, E.E. (1999) Practitioner, researcher, and gender conflict in a qualitative study. *Qualitative Health Research.* 9(4): 455–67.

Hardy, S., Gregory, S., Ramjeet, J. (2009) An exploration of intent for narrative methods of inquiry. *Researcher.* 16(4): 7–19.

Hart, E., Bond, M. (1995) *Action Research for Health and Social Care: A Guide to Practice.* Buckingham: Open University Press.

Health Service Executive. (2008) *Review of Research Ethics Committees in Republic of Ireland.* Dublin: Health Service Executive.

Hearnshaw, H. (2004). Comparison of requirements of research ethics committees in 11 European countries for a non-invasive interventional study. *British Medical Journal.* 328 (7432): 140–1.

Hek, G., Moule, P. (2006) *Making Sense of Research: An Introduction for Health and Social Care Practitioners*, 3rd edn. London: Sage.

Hellweg, S., Johannes, S. (2008) Physiotherapy after traumatic brain injury: a systematic review of the literature. *Brain Injury.* 22(5): 365–73.

Holloway I., Wheeler S. (2010) *Qualitative Research in Nursing and Healthcare*, 3rd edn. Oxford: Blackwell.

Hutchinson, A.M., Johnston, L. (2004) Bridging the divide: a survey of nurses' opinions regarding barriers to, and facilitators of, research utilization in the practice setting. *Journal of Clinical Nursing.* 13: 304–15.

Johnson, M. (2002) The medication adherence model: a guide for assessing medication taking. *Research and Theory for Nursing Practice: An International Journal.* 16(3): 179–92.

Johnson, N., Taylor, R. (2014) Using research and evidence in practice. In Taylor, R. (ed.), *The Essentials of Nursing and Healthcare Research.* Sage: London.

Jones, M., Rattray, J. (2010) Questionnaire design. In Gerrish, K., Lacey, A. (eds) *The Research Process in Nursing*, 6th edn. Oxford: Wiley-Blackwell. pp. 369–81.

Katz, J. (1972) *Experimentation with Human Beings.* Available at: www.columbia.edu/itc/history/rothman/COL476I5027.pdf (accessed 8 April 2013).

Kenny, D.J. (2005) Nurses' use of research in practice at three US army hospitals. *Nursing Leadership.* 18(3): 45–67.

Kleinman, A. (1988) *The Illness Narratives: Suffering, Healing and the Human Condition.* NewYork: Basic Books.

Knight, P. (2002) *Small Scale Research.* London: Sage.

Koball, H.L., Moiduddin, E., Henderson, J., Goesling, B., Besculides, M. (2010) What do we know about the link between marriage and health? *Journal of Family Issues.* 31(8): 1019–40.

Kocaman, G., Seren, S., Lash, A.A., Kurt, S., Bengu, N., Yurumezoglu, H.A. (2010) Barriers to research utilisation by staff nurses in a university hospital. *Journal of Clinical Nursing.* 19: 1908–18.

Kuhn, T. (1970) *The Structure of Scientific Revolutions*, 2nd edn. Chicago: University of Chicago Press.

Lahlafi, A. (2007) Conducting a literature review: how to carry out bibliographical database searches. *British Journal of Cardiac Nursing*, 2(12): 566–9.

Lauzon Clabo, L.M. (2008) An ethnography of pain assessment and the role of social context on two postoperative units. *Journal of Advanced Nursing.* 61(5): 531–9.

Lee, P. (2006) Understanding and critiquing quantitative research papers. *Nursing Times.* 102(28): 28–30.

Lincoln, Y.S., Guba, E. (1985) *Naturalistic Inquiry.* Thousand Oaks, CA: Sage.

Lynn, M.R. (1986) Determination and quantification of content validity. *Nurse Researcher.* 35(6): 383–5.

Lyons, C., Brown, T., Tseng, M.H., Casey, J., McDonald, R. (2011) Evidence-based practice and research utilisation: perceived research knowledge, attitudes, practices, and barriers among Australian paediatric occupational therapists. *Australian Occupational Therapy Journal.* 58: 178–86.

Madon, T., Hofman, K.J., Kupfer, L., Glass, R.I. (2007) Public health: implementation science. *Science.* 318(5857): 1728–9.

Mansell, J. (2011) *Structured Observational Research in Services for People with Learning Disabilities.* School for Social Care Research (SSCR) methods review, 10. London: National Institute for Health Research (NIHR) School for Social Care Research.

Mays, N., Pope, C. (1995) Rigour and qualitative research. *British Medical Journal.* 311: 109–12.

McCambridge, J., Witton, J., Elbourne, D.R. (2014) Systematic review of the Hawthorne effect: new concepts are needed to study research participation effects. *Journal of Clinical Epidemiology.* 67: 267–77.

McDermot, B.E. (2013) Coercion in research: are prisoners the only vulnerable population? *Journal of the American Academy of Psychiatry and the Law.* 41: 8–13.

McHugh, M.L. (2012) Interrater reliability: the kappa statistic. *Biochemica Medica.* 22(3): 276–82.

McKenna, H., Hasson, F., Keeney, S. (2010) Surveys. In Gerrish, K., Lacey, A. (eds), *The Research Process in Nursing.* 6th edn. Oxford: Wiley-Blackwell. pp. 216–26.

McKeown, E., Nelson, S., Anderson, J., Low, N., Elford, J. (2010) Disclosure, discrimination and desire: experiences of Black and South Asian gay men in Britain. *Culture, Health & Sexuality.* 12(7): 843–56.

McMahon, S., Fleury, J. (2012) External validity of physical activity interventions for community dwelling older adults with fall risk: a quantitative systematic literature review. *Journal of Advanced Nursing.* 68(10): 2140–54.

Meho, L.I. (2006) E-mail interviewing in qualitative research: a methodological discussion. *Journal of the American Society for Information Science and Technology.* 57(10): 1284–95.

Meyer, J. (2010) Action research. In Gerrish, K., Lacey, A. (eds), *The Research Process in Nursing,* 6th edn. Oxford: Wiley-Blackwell. pp. 257–70.

Meyer, P.J. (2003) *What Would You do if You Knew You Couldn't Fail? Creating SMART Goals: Attitude is Everything if You Want to Succeed Above and Beyond.* Scotts Valley, CA: Meyer Resource Group Incorporated.

Miller, F., Brody, H. (2007) Clinical equipoise and the incoherence of research ethics. *Journal of Medicine & Philosophy.* 32: 151–65.

Milner, M.F., Estabrooks, C.A., Humphrey, C. (2005) Clinical nurse educators as agents for change: increasing research utilization. *International Journal of Nursing Studies.* 42(8): 899–914.

Milner, M., Estabrooks, C.A., Myrick, F. (2006) Research utilization and clinical nurse educators: a systematic review. *Journal of Evaluation in Clinical Practice.* 12(6): 639–55.

Moreno-Casbas, T., Fuentelsaz-Gallego, C., Gil de Miguel, A., Gonzalez-Maria, E., Clarke, S.P. (2011) Spanish nurses' attitudes towards research and perceived barriers and facilitators of research utilization: a comparative survey of nurses with or without experiences as principal investigators. *Journal of Clinical Nursing.* 20: 1936–47.

Moule, P., Goodman, M. (2014) *Nursing Research: An Introduction,* 2nd edn. Los Angeles: Sage.

Muir Gray, J.A. (2001) *Evidence-based Health Care.* Edinburgh: Churchill Livingstone.

Muldoon, K., Biesty, L., Smith, V. (2014) 'I found the OSCE very stressful': Student midwives' attitudes towards an objective-structured clinical examination (OSCE). *Nurse Education Today.* 34: 468–73.

Murch, S. (2009) Separating inflammation from speculation. *Lancet.* 362 (9394): 1498–9.

Neergaard, M.A., Olesen, F. Rikke, S., Andersen, R., Sondergaard, J. (2009) Qualitative description – the poor cousin of health research? *BMC Medical Research Methodology.* 9(52). Available at: www.biomedcentral.com/1471-2288/9/52.

Newell, R., Burnard, P. (2011) *Research for Evidenced-based Practice in Healthcare,* 2nd edn. Oxford: Wiley-Blackwell.

Noble, R. (2007). *Introduction to Medical Ethics: Medical Ethics in the Global Village.* London: Centre for Reproductive Ethics and Rights, University College London.

Norlyk, A., Harder, I. (2010) What makes a phenomenological study phenomenological? An analysis of peer-reviewed empirical nursing studies. *Qualitative Health Research.* 20(3): 420–31.

Office of NIH History. (1996) *Dr. Joseph Goldberger and the War on Pellagra.* Available at: http://history.nih.gov/exhibits/goldberger/index.html (accessed 30 August 2013).

Ohio Nurses Organisation. (2013) What do I know? Ethical dilemmas in nursing and health. *Indiana State Nurses Association Bulletin.* Feb–Mar: 5–12.

Overcash, J.A. (2003) Narrative research: a review of methodology and relevance to clinical practice. *Critical Reviews in Oncology/Hematology.* 48: 179–84.

Overy, R. (2011) Nuremberg: Nazis on trial. Available at: www.bbc.co.uk/history/worldwars/wwtwo/nuremberg_article_01.shtml(accessed 5 May 2014).

Paley, J., Eva, G. (2005) Narrative vigilance: the analysis of stories in health care. *Nursing Philosophy.* 6: 83–97.

Parahoo, K. (2000) Barriers to, and facilitators of, research utilization among nurses in Northern Ireland. *Journal of Advanced Nursing.* 31(1): 89–98.

Parahoo, K. (2006) *Nursing Research: Principles, Process and Issues*, 2nd edn. Houndmills: Palgrave Macmillan.

Paterson, B.L. (2001) Refining your research question. *The Canadian Nurse*. 97(2): 12–13.

Payne, C., Mason, B. (1998) Autism, inflammatory bowel disease and MMR vaccine. *Lancet*. 351: 907.

Pinkerton, C.R. (2002) Ethical approval for multicentre clinical trials in children: contrasting systems in three European countries. *European Journal of Cancer*. 38(8): 1051–8.

Polit, D.F., Beck, C.T. (2012) *Nursing Research: Generating and Assessing Evidence for Nursing Practice*, 9th edn. Philadelphia: Wolters Kluwer Health/ Lippincott Williams & Wilkins.

Polit, D.F., Beck, C.T. (2014) *Essentials of Nursing Research: Appraising Evidence for Nursing Practice*, 8th edn. Philadelphia: Wolters Kluwer Health/ Lippincott Williams & Wilkins.

Polit, D.F., Northam, S. (2011) Impact factors in nursing journals. *Nursing Outlook*. 59: 18–28.

Profetto-McGrath, J., Hesketh, K.L., Lang, S., Estabrooks, C.A. (2003) A study of critical thinking and research utilization among nurses. *Western Journal of Nursing Research*. 25(3): 322–37.

Rebar, C., Gersch, C., MacNee, C., McCabe, S. (2011) *Understanding Nursing Research: Using Research in Evidence-based Practice*, 3rd edn. Philadelphia: Wolters Kluwer/ Lippincott Williams & Wilkins.

Reason, P., Bradbury, H. (2008) *Handbook of Action Research: Participative Inquiry and Practice*, 2nd edn. London: Sage.

Robinson, W.M., Unruh, B.T. (2008) Chapter 7: The hepatitis experiments at the Willowbrook state school. In Emanual, E.J., Grady, C., Crouch, R.A., Lie, R., Miller, F.G., Wendler, D. (eds), *The Oxford Textbook of Clinical Research Ethics*. Oxford; Oxford University Press. pp. 80–85.

Robson, C. (2011) *Real World Research*, 3rd edn. Oxford: Blackwell.

Rodgers, B.L., Knafl, K.A. (2000) *Concept Development in Nursing*, 2nd edn. Philadelphia: Saunders.

Rogers, E. (2003) *Diffusion of Innovations*, 5th edn. New York: Free Press.

Rolfe, G. (1999) Insufficient evidence: the problems of evidence-based medicine. *Nurse Education Today*. 19: 422–42.

Rolfe, G. (2006). Validity, trustworthiness and rigour: quality and the idea of qualitative research. *Journal of Advanced Nursing*. 53(3): 304–10.

Rolfe, G., Gardner, L. (2006) Towards a geology of evidence-based practice – A discussion paper. *International Journal of Nursing Studies*. 43: 903–13.

Ross, T. (2012) *A Survival Guide for Health Research Methods*. Maidenhead: Open University Press.

Rossman, B., Engstrom, J.L., Meier, P.P. (2012) Healthcare providers' perspectives of breast feeding peer counsellors in the neonatal intensive care unit. *Research in Nursing & Health*. 35: 460–74.

Rothman, D. (1982) Were Tuskegee & Willowbrook 'studies in nature'? Available at: http://columbiauniversity.net/itc/history/rothman/COL479E4711.pdf (accessed 8 February 2014).

Routledge, F.S. (2007) Exploring the use of feminist philosophy within nursing research to enhance post-positivist methodologies in the study of cardiovascular health. *Nursing Philosophy*. 8: 278–90.

Ryan, F., Coughlan, M., Cronin, P. (2007) Step-by-step guide to critiquing research. Part 2: qualitative research. *British Journal of Nursing*. 16(12): 738–44.

Ryan, F., Coughlan, M., Cronin, P. (2009) Interviewing in qualitative research: the one-to-one interview. *International Journal of Therapy and Rehabilitation*. 16(6): 309–14.

Sackett, D.L., Rosenberg, W.M.C., Muir Gray, J.A., Haynes, R.B., Scott Richardson, W. (1996) Evidence-based medicine: what it is and what it isn't. *British Medical Journal*. 312 (7023): 71.

Sadler, G.R., Lee, H.C., Lim, R.S., Fullerton, J. (2010) Recruitment of hard-to-reach population subgroups via adaptations of the snowball sampling strategy. *Nursing & Health
Sciences*. 12: 369–74.

Saha, S., Saint, S., Christakis, D.A. (2003) Impact factor: a valid measure of journal quality?
Journal Medical Library Association. 91(1): 42–6.

Sandelowski, M. (2000) Whatever happened to qualitative description? *Research in Nursing
& Health*. 23(4): 334–40.

Sandelowski, M. (2003) Rigor or rigor mortis: the problem of rigor in qualitative research
revisited. *Advanced Nursing Science*. 16(2): 1–8.

Schoenborn, C.A. (2004) Marital status and health: United States, 1999–2002. *Advance Data*.
No. 351. Available at: www.cdc.gov/nchs/data/ad/ad351.pdf

Scottish Intercollegiate Guidelines (2013) *Methodology Checklist 1: Systematic Reviews and
Meta-analysis*. Available at www.sign.ac.uk/methodology/checklists.html

Shea, B.J., Grimshaw, J.M., Wells, G.A., Boer, S.M., Andersson, N., Hamel, C., Ashley, C.,
Porter, A.C., Tugwell, P., Moher, D., Bouter, L.M. (2007) Development of AMSTAR: a
measurement tool to assess the methodological quality of systematic reviews. *BMC Medical
Research Methodology*, 7: 10. doi:10.1186/1471-2288-7-10

Shea, J., Klainin-Yobas, P. Mackey, S. (2013) Young Singaporean women's knowledge of cervical
cancer and pap smear screening: a descriptive study. *Journal of Clinical Nursing* 22(23–24):
3310–19.

Sheach Leith, V.M. (2007) Consent and nothing but consent? The organ retention scandal.
Sociology of Health and Illness. 29(7): 1023–42.

Shenton, A.K. (2004) Strategies for ensuring trustworthiness in qualitative research projects.
Education for information. 22: 63–75.

Simons, L., Lathlean, J. (2010) Mixed methods. In: Gerrish, K., Lacey, A. (eds) *The Research
Process in Nursing*, 6th edn. Wiley-Blackwell: Chichester. pp. 331–42.

Skårderud, F. (2007) Shame and pride in anorexia nervosa: a qualitative descriptive study.
European Eating Disorders Review. 15: 81–97.

Sleep, J., Grant, A., Garcia, J., Elbourne, D., Spencer, J., Chalmers, I. (1984) West Berkshire
perineal management trial. *British Medical Journal*. 289: 587–90.

Smith, V., Begley, C., Devane, D. (2014) Detection and management of decreased fetal movements
in Ireland: a national survey of midwives' and obstetricians' practices. *Midwifery*. 30: 43–9.

Smith, V., Devane, D., Higgins, S. (2011) Practices for predicting and preventing preterm birth
in Ireland: a national survey. *Irish Journal of Medical Science*. 180: 63–7.

Smith, V., Devane, D., Murphy-Lawless, J. (2012) Risk in maternity care: a concept analysis.
International Journal of Childbirth. 2(2): 126–35.

Spradley, J. (1979) *The Ethnographic Interview*. New York: Holt, Rinehart and Winston.

Squire, P. (1988) Why the 1936 Literary Digest Poll failed. *Public Opinion Quarterly*. 52(1):
125–33.

Squires, J.E., Hutchinson, A.M., Bostrom, A., O'Rourke, H.M., Cobban, S.J., Estabrooks,
C.A. (2011) To what extent do nurses use research in clinical practice? A systematic review.
Implementation Science. 6(21): 1–18.

Stake, R.E. (2005) Qualitative case studies. In Denzin, N.K, Lincoln, Y.S. (eds), *Handbook of
Qualitative Research*, 3rd edn. Thousand Oaks, CA: Sage. pp. 443–66.

Steup, M. (2012) *Epistemology. The Stanford Encyclopedia of Philosophy* (Winter 2012
Edition), Edward N. Zalta (ed.). Available at: http://plato.stanford.edu/archives/win2012/
entries/epistemology/

Streubert, H.J., Carpenter, D.R. (2011) *Qualitative Research in Nursing: Advancing the
Humanistic Imperative*, 5th edn. Philadelphia: Wolters Kluwer Health/Lippincott Williams
& Wilkins.

Sword, W., Heaman, M.I., Brooks, S., Tough, S., Janssen, P.A., Young, D., Kingston, D.,
Helewa, M.E., Akhtar-Danesh, N., Hutton, E. (2012) Women's and care providers'

perspectives of quality prenatal care: a qualitative descriptive study. *BMC Pregnancy and Childbirth*. 12(29): 1–18.

The Liberty Guide to Human Rights. (2009) *Definition of Personal Data and Personal Sensitive Data*. Available at: www.yourrights.org.uk (accessed 3 October 2013).

Thompson, D.S., O'Leary, K., Jensen, E., Scott,-Findlay, S., O'Brien-Pallas, L., Estabrooks, C.A. (2008) The relationship between busyness and research utilization: it is about time. *Journal of Clinical Nursing*. 17: 539–48.

Tobin, G.A., Begley, C.M. (2004) Methodological rigour within a qualitative framework. *Journal of Advanced Nursing*. 48(4): 385–96.

Torraco, R.J. (2005) Writing integrative literature reviews: guidelines and examples. *Human Resource Development Review*. 4(3): 356–67.

Tully, J. (2000) The new system of review by multicentre research ethics committees: prospective study. *British Medical Journal*. 320(7243): 1179–82.

Tuskegee University (2013) *About the USPHS Syphilis Study*. Available at: www.tuskegee. edu/about_us/centers_of_excellence/bioethics_center/about_the_usphs_syphilis_study. aspx (accessed 8 April 2013).

Wakefield, A.J., Murch, S.H., Anthony, A., Linnell, J., Casson, D.M., Malik, M., Berelowitz, M., Dhillon, A.P., Thomson, M.A., Harvey, P., Valentine, A., Davies, S.E., Walker-Smith, J.A. (1998) Ileal lymphoid hyperplasia, non-specific colitis, and pervasive developmental disorder in children [retracted]. *Lancet*. 351: 637–41.

Walker, L., Avant, K. (2011) *Strategies for Theory Construction in Nursing*, 5th edn. Norwalk: Appleton and Lange.

Wangansteen, S., Johansson, I.S., Björkström, M.E., Nordström, G. (2011) Research utilisation and critical thinking among newly graduated nurses: predictors for research use. A quantitative cross-sectional study. *Journal of Clinical Nursing*. 20: 2436–47.

Watson, H., Booth, J., Whyte, R. (2010) Observation. In Gerrish, K., Lacey, A. (eds), *The Research Process in Nursing*, 6th edn. Oxford: Wiley-Blackwell. pp. 382–94.

Weijer, C., Shapiro, S., Cranley-Glass, K. (2000) Clinical equipoise and not the uncertainty principle is the moral underpinning of the randomised controlled trial. *BMJ: British Medical Journal*. 321: 756–8.

Wells, G.A., Shea, B., O'Connell, D., Peterson, J., Welch, V., Losos, M., Tugwell, P. (2014) The Newcastle-Ottawa Scale (NOS) for assessing the quality of nonrandomised studies in meta-analyses. Available at: www.ohri.ca (accessed 4 April 2014).

Wells, M. (2009) Surveying the experience of living with metastatic breast cancer: comparing face-to-face and online recruitment (paper 578). *Journal of Research in Nursing*. 14: 57–9.

Whittemore, R., Knafl, K. (2005) The integrative review: updated methodology. *Journal of Advanced Nursing*. 52(5): 546–53.

Williams, A.F., Manias, E., Walker, R. (2008) Adherence to multiple, prescribed medications in diabetic kidney disease: a qualitative study of consumers' and health professionals' perspectives. *International Journal of Nursing Studies*. 45: 1742–56.

Wood, M.J., Ross-Kerr, J.C. (2006) *Basic Steps in Planning Nursing Research*, 6th edn. Burlington, MA: Jones and Bartlett Publishers.

World Health Organization. (2001) *International Classification of Functioning, Disability and Health: ICF*. Geneva: World Health Organization (WHO).

World Health Organization. (2009) *Research Ethics Committees: Basic Concepts for Capacity Building*. Geneva: World Health Organization (WHO).

World Health Organization. (2011) *Standards and Operational Guidance for Ethics Review of Health-related Research with Human Participants*. Geneva: World Health Organization (WHO).

Yin, R.E. (2013) *Case Study Research Design and Methods*, 5th edn. London: Sage.

Index